National Academy Press

The National Academy Press was created by the National Academy of
Sciences to publish the reports issued by the Academy and by the
National Academy of Engineering, the Institute of Medicine, and the
National Research Council, all operating under the charter granted to
the National Academy of Sciences by the Congress of the United States.

The New Health Care for Profit

Doctors and Hospitals in a Competitive Environment

Edited by Bradford H. Gray

Institute of Medicine

NATIONAL ACADEMY PRESS
Washington, D.C.   1983

The Institute of Medicine was chartered in 1970 by the National Academy of Sciences to enlist distinguished members of the appropriate professions in the examination of policy matters pertaining to the health of the public. In this, the Institute acts under both the Academy's 1863 congressional charter responsibility to be an adviser to the federal government and its own initiative in identifying issues of medical care, research, and education.

Publication IOM 83-001

Library of Congress Cataloging in Publication Data

Main entry under title:

The new health care for profit.

1. Health facilities, Proprietary—United States.
2. Medical corporations—United States. I. Gray,
Bradford H., 1942–   II. Institute of Medicine
(U.S.) [DNLM: 1. Delivery of health care—Trends—
United States. 2. Economics, Hospital—Trends—United
States. 3. Economics, Medical—Trends—United States.
4. Ethics, Medical—United States. 5. Financial
management—Trends—United States. 6. Hospitals—Trends
—United States. WX 157 N532]
RA981.A2N48   1983   362.1'1'0973   83-8054
ISBN 0-309-03377-2

Available from

NATIONAL ACADEMY PRESS
2101 Constitution Avenue, NW
Washington, DC 20418

Printed in the United States of America

Preface

The papers in this volume grew out of a series of informal discussions and activities going back to June 1981, when the Institute of Medicine brought together a diverse group of knowledgeable persons for a one-day workshop titled "Trends in For-Profit Health Care." The workshop was organized by Carleton Evans, M.D., then Director of the Division of Health Care Services at the Institute, and was supported by National Academy of Sciences' program initiation funds. The workshop and the subsequent discussions resulted in a plan for a two-year study of physician involvement in for-profit enterprise in health care, to be completed at the end of 1984. A preliminary phase of the Institute's study, during which this collection of papers was prepared, was supported by the Hospital Corporation of America and the Commonwealth Fund.

We would like to thank the following members of the Institute's Board on Health Care Services and the Institute's Council for reviewing various of the papers published herein: Linda Aiken, Richard Edgahl, Charles Lewis, Peter Libassi, David Mechanic, Howard Newman, and Sam Shapiro.

Karl D. Yordy, *Director*
Division of Health Care Services

Contents

The New Health Care for Profit

Doctors and Hospitals in a Competitive Environment

An Introduction to the New Health Care for Profit

Bradford H. Gray

With little initial public notice, a vigorous and varied for-profit sector has developed in the predominantly not-for-profit world of medical care. Health services are now being provided by thousands of for-profit organizations that range from large investor-owned hospital and nursing home chains, whose stock has rapidly appreciated on the New York Stock Exchange, to various types of independent medical facilities—such as ambulatory surgery centers, cardiopulmonary testing centers, etc.—owned by local investors who often are also physicians. Sometimes the physician-owners generate revenues for the facilities by referring patients for services.

Health care has long included a mixture of for-profit and not-for-profit activities. The manufacture and marketing of pharmaceuticals and medical equipment have always been predominantly organized on a for-profit basis. The health insurance industry has included both for-profit and not-for-profit organizations. Not-for-profit forms have been more typical of the organizations that provide medical services to patients. This is because of the origins and evolution of the hospital as a charity institution providing care to the poor and not because of any organized social policy decision regarding appropriateness of dif-

I would like to acknowledge the contribution of Carl Evans to a preliminary paper from which part of this paper was developed and to thank Helen Darling and Karl Yordy for their comments and suggestions on drafts.

1

ferent organizational forms. The availability and predictability of revenues that came with the rise of large-scale governmental payment for health services has opened up profit-making opportunities that did not previously exist.

The rapid growth of for-profit corporations as direct providers of health services represents an appreciable shift on medicine's business side; the new investor-owned health care companies are to the old "doctor's hospitals" what agribusiness is to the family farm. In an earlier era, many communities were served by doctor-owned hospitals, usually in rural America, and the arrangement was open and accepted by custom. Cities more often were served by larger voluntary or public hospitals, but even there physicians' proprietary hospitals were not unheard of. (An interesting and largely unrecognized aspect of the growth of the large proprietary chains in the past decade is that it has apparently decreased the amount of direct physician ownership and entrepreneurial control of hospitals.) Some physicians also have owned pharmacies, laboratories, and radiology units and have engaged in specialty referral networks and self-referral. Although largely accepted by the public, some of these practices have from time to time been scrutinized by the profession because they raise concerns about such matters as conflict of interest in patient care decisions.

The exact dimensions of the for-profit sector of providers of health services are not known. Rough estimates have put the gross revenues of investor-owned health care industry as high as $40 billion.[1] Observers of the industry agree that it continues to expand, encouraged in part by federal reimbursement practices under Medicare and by other features of the American health care system that have created, perhaps inadvertently, a highly favorable environment for growth.

In 1982 about 10 percent of U.S. hospitals were owned by the for-profit hospital chains, and another 4 percent were managed by those firms.[2] Another 5 percent of U.S. hospitals were independently owned proprietary hospitals. The number of hospitals owned or managed by for-profit hospital chains (i.e., those owning at least 3 hospitals) almost doubled between 1976 and 1982 (from 533 to 1,040 hospitals), a period in which the total number of hospitals in the United States decreased slightly and the number of independently owned for-profit hospitals declined rapidly (many being purchased by the chains).[3] Most of the firms that own chains of hospitals (as well as those that own other kinds of health service facilities) were established only in the last 15 years. They have grown by means of the purchase, construction, and contract management of institutions and by buying smaller chains. The growing size of the companies has itself attracted attention. As one observer graphically described the largest merger to date:

The announcement early in 1981 that Hospital Corporation of America had acquired Hospital Affiliates International, formerly a property of the Insurance Company of North America, projected a $2 billion corporate giant in the hospital field and caused a flurry of excitement tinged with anxiety in the medical-hospital establishment. . . . The new corporation would have five percent of all the beds and two percent of all the money, give or take, and that was enough to make a lot of people look around and say, "What's going on here?"[4]

For-profit organizations are more numerous among other types of health care facilities than among hospitals. More than three-quarters of nursing homes are proprietary,[5] and about 40 percent of hemodialysis in this country is provided by profit-making units.[6] For-profit organizations now provide emergency medical services, home care, mobile CAT scanning, cardiopulmonary testing, industrial health screening, rehabilitation counseling, dental care, weight control clinics, alcohol and drug abuse programs, comprehensive prepaid HMO programs, and laboratory and related services. An example of the proliferation of specialized for-profit health care organization is the existence of a trade association for "urgent care centers," which are estimated to number 500 to 600.[7]

Some analogous changes are also taking place in the not-for-profit health care sector. Not-for-profit health institutions (the survival of which also requires an excess of revenues over expenses) have variously been forming chains, establishing for-profit subsidiaries, selling services to other hospitals for profit, and taking on other attributes of the for-profit enterprises. There has been at least a short-term boom in the activities of attorneys and accountants who advise on reorganizing and incorporating various services to maximize revenues and reduce taxes.[8] Even the language used today in hospital journals—such as "lines of business," "market shares," and "profit centers"—would have seemed foreign in the health policy world of only a few years ago.

The Changing Health Care Environment

The recent surge in for-profit activity in health care has occurred during a period of rapid growth in national expenditures for health care. However, this environment is changing. Although such expenditures will undoubtedly continue to increase, serious efforts are under way, both in government and in the private sector, to constrain this growth. This intensifying squeeze on money for health care, in combination with the growing supply of physicians, is heightening competition among hospitals, other health care facilities, and physicians for capital and for patients who are adequately insured. This new competitive environment is developing independently of policies and proposals explicitly intended to make health care more competitive, although the adoption of such proposals reinforces the trend.

Since this struggle for resources threatens the survival of some institutions and the incomes of physicians, powerful incentives are created for changing past ways of doing business. There has been, for example, a visible increase in attention to such ideas as strategic planning, more aggressive marketing techniques, vertical and horizontal integration, improving efficiency, generating new sources of revenues and protecting old ones, and using various other business practices that evince dedication to the generation of profits or surpluses, "the bottom line." Many of the consequences of this competition seem healthy and beneficial—e.g., making more efficient use of resources. Other consequences may affect the future well-being of such important activities as graduate medical education, research, and care of indigent patients that have been at least partially subsidized through revenues from paying patients. This changing atmosphere may also have important implications regarding the plausibility of the beliefs and assumptions that have given patients the confidence to entrust their well-being to physicians and that have led society to vest control of a vital component part in a relatively autonomous profession.

The public and its policies and the medical professionals and their institutions may be quite unprepared for many of these new developments. All social institutions—the family, the church, government, medicine—exist within a framework of values, beliefs, and assumptions about the way things are and the way they should be. In relatively stable times, dominant values and beliefs may be so consonant with our social institutions as to be almost imperceptible, let alone questioned. But in times of rapid change and stress we become more aware of the consensual footing on which intricate social arrangements and trust relationships rest, and perhaps find that old values, beliefs, and assumptions are outmoded.

Future government policies regarding health care will be substantially affected by assumptions about such matters as the nature of health care and the responsibilities and behavior of medical professionals and institutions. Much health policy has been predicated on beliefs that the physician follows a different ethic than does the businessman and that hospitals have a mission of service that transcends at least short-term considerations of profitability. As recently expressed by Paul Starr,

The contradiction between professionalism and the rule of the market is long-standing and unavoidable. Medicine and other professions have historically distinguished themselves from business and trade by claiming to be above the market and pure commercialism. In justifying the public's trust, professionals have set higher standards of conduct for themselves than the minimal rules governing the marketplace and maintained that they can be judged under those standards by each other, not by laymen. . . . [The] shift from clients to colleagues in the orientation of work, which professionalism demands, represents a clear departure from the normal rule of the market.[9]

Thus, the growth of the for-profit sector in health care provides a reason to reconsider the assumptions on which so much of our health policy has rested.

Professional Autonomy, Trust, and Health Policy

Our entire health care system is organized largely to carry out decisions made by highly autonomous and independent physicians. Hospitals, for example, are organized to respond to physicians' decisions—even implementing them when the physicians are not physically present. Many aspects of our health care system rest on an assumption that the physician's primary concern is with the needs and care of the patient. Assumptions about motivations—e.g., about whether the physician or hospital primarily seeks to provide needed services or to maximize revenues—must affect the degree of trust between doctor and patient and between society and the medical profession (including the organizations within which physicians practice). In part because the science and technology of medicine are complex and often changing, nonphysicians have tended to leave to the medical profession such matters as criteria or standards for licensure, certification, curriculum development, quality assurance, and academic or institutional accreditation. All of these arrangements reflect high public trust in the medical profession. The strength of this trust arguably will affect all other matters in health care—the behavior of medical institutions; the distribution, utilization, and cost of services; future regulatory strategies in health care; and even patient outcomes.

Trust can take different forms or have different origins.[10] One form of trust is based on perceptions of technical competence. Our willingness to take medications, undergo total anesthesia, or submit to surgery stems largely from trust in the technical competence of the physician, anesthesiologist, or surgeon. A second kind of trust, which also characterizes the doctor-patient relationship and is perhaps necessary to it, involves the expectation of fiduciary obligation or responsibility. Not only do we trust the physician's competence, but we also trust that decisions about our care will be based on our needs not on the physician's desire, for example, for additional income. Although the patient who is in pain and distress has a strong and understandable need to trust the physician, it is easy to see how perceptions of conflict of interest could diminish trust in a physician as one's fiduciary. (However, conflict of interest appears less likely to affect our trust in the technical competence of physicians than it is to influence our trust in their fiduciary role; e.g., some people needing hemodialysis in kidney failure might be most comfortable in a center owned by their physician, on the assumption that there would be better quality control in such a center.)

As individual persons and as a society, we behave differently according to our willingness to trust. Some social arrangements rely heavily on trust. Although this has clear benefits in many instances, a trusting party may be vulnerable to abuse. Certain forms of distrust can serve some of the same functions as trust in facilitating social interaction and exchange.[11] Even when conflicting interests are perceived by the parties, transactions can occur readily. Typically, however, they will rest on a greater exchange of information, on contractual assurances, on legally defined obligations, and so forth. Distrust forms one basis for imposing governmental or regulatory controls. Second opinions about surgery are mechanisms for dealing with distrust (in both the fiduciary and/or the technical competence sense) of physicians. U.S. Food and Drug Administration regulations requiring proof of the safety and efficacy of drugs are mechanisms for the expression of distrust (or, at least, of limited trust) in the technical competence of medical practitioners to decide what drugs to give to patients under what circumstances. Distrust may also lead patients to seek independent sources of information or to seek help from outside the health care system. The behavior that results from distrust may be seen as desirable or undesirable.

Sociological analyses of professions—of which medicine was seen as the prototype—long gave prominence to a "collectivity or service orientation" as a basic defining characteristic of professions.[12] The idea was that physicians, notwithstanding their need to make a living, would put their patients' interests before their own. Indeed, this was the image that the medical profession projected of itself. "A profession," stated the American Medical Association's code of ethics in the first half of the twentieth century, "has for its prime object the service it can render to humanity; reward or financial gain should be a subordinate consideration."[13]

The service ethic is the object of more skepticism today. It has, for example, been described as a "myth created and perpetuated by professionals to enhance their status and to 'silence the critics of monopoly, privilege, and power to which professionals are attempting to cling.' "[14] There are indications that a more profit-oriented or businesslike orientation has developed among physicians. This orientation takes many forms—creating "professional corporations," under the stimulus of tax law changes, for the practice of medicine; moving toward commercial activities, such as advertising, that once were considered unethical; entering into incentive compensation arrangements with medical institutions, such as renting office space from a hospital at a price dependent on the volume of hospital business the physician generates; and establishing or working for profit-making entities for provision of health services. The service ethic is regarded by some critics as an empty ideology from which the medical profession, having persuaded society to accept, gains benefits in prestige and autonomy. Such skepticism is influencing health policy in such ways as regulatory efforts to change physicians' patient care decisions by modifying the economic incentives to which they are seen as responding.

Our dominant medical institutions—hospitals—have their origins in charity and local government and have long been seen as existing primarily to serve a public interest.[15] Nonprofit hospitals benefited from tax exemptions and had public funds and charitable donations as the primary sources of money for construction. Hospitals were seen by many as following a distinct ethic: "Some business men will say that any institution that is not self-supporting should go out of business, but the hospital cannot do this, if it is a good hospital. Its obligation to its community is not measured by its net earnings, but by the service it renders, regardless of whether the community pays for such service or not."[16] Today's authors are more likely to emphasize that the hospital should pay attention to its bottom line than to suggest that hospitals should somehow provide services for which no one will pay. After all, an institution that does not attend to its own financial requirements will cease to exist to serve any larger public interest.

Earlier in the twentieth century the hospital became the means of organizing and centralizing the technologies needed for the modern physician to practice medicine. However, the relationship between hospitals and physicians is changing. Today, hospitals are increasingly defining their own institutional goals, which may include an emphasis on making a revenue surplus or profit, and physicians are increasingly the objects of systematic and well-planned marketing efforts.[17] A marketing strategy may identify both the physicians (and, therefore, the patients) to whom the hospital wants to appeal and the physicians and patients whom the hospital wants to avoid. The relationship between hospitals and physicians—in terms of both economic arrangements and institutional governance—are in flux as hospitals are reorganized or get new owners. Furthermore, the current move to reimburse hospitals on the basis of prospectively set, per case rates creates new incentives for hospitals to attempt to influence or control physicians' patient care decisions.

Thus, there are many reasons to believe that our health care system is moving into a distinctively new phase. The relationship between hospitals and physicians increasingly is being seen in terms of the exercise of power and competition for scarce resources.[18] The primary source of physicians' power is their control of patients—deciding what services they need and who should provide those services. A second source of power stems from the increasing willingness of physicians to enter into direct competition with hospitals for certain types of patients—a development seen, for example, in the growth of physician-owned ambulatory surgery centers. However, hospitals, particularly those that are part of a chain, are not without their own sources of power in relation to physicians. One is the growing number of physicians, which increases their competitiveness with each other. Another is that the career advancement and authority of a hospital administrator in a chain are to some extent external to the local community and its physicians, although success at the local level will continue to depend substantially on the administrator's ability to work with local physicians and other interested citizens.

Implications of the Current Changes in For-Profit Health Care

The implications of the trends in for-profit enterprise in health care are not yet clear, although they already are very controversial. Some see the trends in for-profit enterprise as bringing a degree of rationality and discipline to the management of a health care system that has seldom been under rational control or sound management. The profit motive and the operation of markets are seen by many as the most efficient way to define and meet human needs in an environment of scarce resources. Furthermore, bringing in the investor opens a whole new source of capital to an increasingly capital-intensive and capital-hungry enterprise. Convincing arguments can be made that there is no rational justification for traditional assumptions that the nonprofit form is best for the health care system.[19]

Those who are less certain about the benefits of a growing for-profit sector in health care raise several types of concerns. Perhaps the most fundamental are those that question how the growth of for-profit health care corporations will affect the ethos and social responsibilities of the medical profession itself, as Relman argued in his article in *The New England Journal of Medicine* on the "medical-industrial complex."[20] These issues include public perceptions of the medical profession, the importance and determinants of trust in the doctor-patient relationship, what it means to be a physician, and arrangements between physicians and the institutions where medical care is provided.

The type of relationship between physicians and medical facilities can cause concern about the possibile contamination of the physician's role as it pertains to the patient. One such situation exists when physicians are employees of an organization and are to some extent subject to organizational control. This is an old concern and has always been somewhat troublesome (as in organized medicine's long-standing opposition to the "corporate practice of medicine"), although there has been little experience to date with physicians as employees of investor-owned medical organizations. Another type of problematic relationship is physician ownership of facilities (hospitals, nursing homes, radiology centers, and the like) to which they make referrals. The physician with an economic stake in the full utilization of a facility has an apparent conflict of interest when evaluating patients' needs for the type of service that the facility provides. Finally, there are situations in which physicians enter into incentive arrangements with institutions such that the institution rewards the physician for making patient care decisions that benefit the institution. One example is the practice of leasing office space to physicians at rates that depend on the number of patients the physician admits to the hospital. Other examples are suggested by one consultant's advice to hospitals:

Hospitals should consider making technical and financial resources available on a joint venture basis to selected members of their medical staffs to further their professional practices. . . . The hospital should not be construed as offering its resources in exchange for physician business through formal contracts. It is far better to offer some types of assistance which, if withdrawn, pose some economic risk to the physician, and to let the performance expected under terms of such an agreement remain implicit, though crystal clear. . . . Hospitals do not need to own or operate their own feeder systems. Through joint ventures [with physicians] they can assure the same result—sustained hospital utilization.[21]

A second set of questions pertains to the effects of the growth of for-profit corporations in health care on other parts of the system, particularly medical research, medical education, and health care for the poor. To an extent that has never been adequately assessed or understood, all of these activities have been subsidized by revenues from the provision of services to paying (or insured) patients who were charged more than the services cost. Types of services or patients that can generate a profit under current reimbursement mechanisms are clearly of interest to the new health care corporations, whose purpose is to return those profits to stockholders or to increase the value of their stock. As such services and patients are taken over by for-profit firms, some observers are concerned about what will happen to research, education, care for the poor, and institutions that have met these needs in part through subsidization. Although successful for-profit firms will pay taxes, there is no reason to assume such revenue would be used to support these functions. Questions also have been raised about the social responsibilities of health care providers (and the extent to which both for-profit and the not-for-profit providers are meeting such responsibilities) and about the soundness of health care policies that depend to an important extent on hidden subsidization to produce desired social benefits.

A final set of questions concerns whether the for-profit institutions are more efficient and less costly. Although some studies have begun to appear[22] and more are under way, comparisons of cost and efficiency in for-profit and not-for-profit health care institutions are difficult to interpret without better information than now exists about costs and productivity in hospitals, the comparability of patient populations served by different institutions, and other ways in which institutions differ.

The Institute of Medicine Project

To begin to address some of these questions, the Institute of Medicine has undertaken an examination of the implications of new arrangements and approaches to earning profits from the provision of health services. This collection of papers is the initial product of that effort. They are being published at the beginning of a two-year study that will describe the ways that physicians are becoming engaged in for-profit health care enterprises; will summarize information about the consequences of physician involvement in different forms of for-profit enterprises; will discuss the functions of "profits" and how these functions are met in not-for-profit organizations; will analyze the public policies and economic forces that are contributing to the growth of for-profit enterprise in health care; and will examine professional and ethical issues in conflict-of-interest, professional autonomy, and public trust.

These papers, which were commissioned as a preliminary step for this study, provide general background for policy studies on the growth and meaning of the for-profit health care sector. The authors of the papers generally have not reached conclusions but have identified and analyzed questions that merit further consideration and have provided information from which such consideration can begin. Although the papers cover a variety of topics, all are related to an important aspect of the trend toward for-profit enterprise, whether expressed in the behavior of organizations or in the behavior of physicians. Three of the papers in this volume are primarily concerned with medical institutions, three are primarily concerned with physicians, and one is on the relationship between physicians and hospitals.

The paper by John F. Horty and Daniel M. Mulholland III describes the legal differences between for-profit and not-for-profit hospitals. These differences include tax exemptions, reimbursement policies, and available sources of capital. In a discussion of strategies that not-for-profit hospitals are using to overcome certain disadvantages resulting from their present organizational form, the authors see these strategies as gradually blurring the differences between not-for-profit and investor-owned hospitals.

Richard B. Siegrist, Jr.'s paper treats a distinctive feature of investor-owned hospital management companies—the fact that their stock is traded on the stock exchange. Siegrist describes the major hospital management firms from the perspective of the investment analysts who follow them. He notes that Wall Street has looked favorably on the hospital management companies, whose stock prices have rapidly appreciated. The analysts cite several major factors as responsible for the performance of these companies, including their access to and use of capital, the stability of their sources of income, the regulatory environment, economies of scale, and management expertise. Siegrist also examines some of the differences among the major companies.

Most hospitals that have been acquired in the past by the investor-owned hospital chains have been locally owned proprietary hospitals, but, because of the dwindling number of independent proprietary hospitals, future acquisitions increasingly will be voluntary and government-owned hospitals. The sale of such a hospital to an investor-owned chain can be a cause of concern within both the community and institution, but little information is now available about the nature of those concerns or how the purchasing company responds to them. In her paper, Jessica Townsend describes the findings from her exploratory case studies of the sale of four hospitals to investor-owned chains. She describes the reactions of people likely to be affected by the sale of a hospital, the process by which the sale was negotiated, and actions that were taken by the buyer to address the concerns of interested parties. Her analysis suggests the range and types of concerns of various parties—hospital administrators, physicians, board members, consumer groups—and points out factors that may influence the satisfactory completion of a sale.

Stephen M. Shortell's paper is primarily concerned with linkage between hospitals and physicians in the important area of hospital decision making. He analyzes the types of organizational decisions that must be made in hospitals and summarizes the literature on physician participation in hospital governance. He speculates on how such participation may vary, depending on whether a hospital is organized on a for-profit or not-for-profit basis and whether the hospital is part of a chain. He also examines a wide range of changes that are taking place in health care today that have implications for institutional decision making and physician involvement therein.

The behavior of physicians is the subject of Harold S. Luft's paper. One of the implicit concerns in the emergence of a more explicit profit-seeking orientation in health care is that physicians' patient care decisions may be affected. A customary expectation among economists is that incentives will affect behavior, but physicians have tended to argue that their patient care decisions are based on patients' needs and the state of biomedical knowledge. Luft, an economist, describes the economist's and physician's perspectives, noting differences in the types of evidence they might use in supporting their positions. He describes evidence regarding the influence of economic incentives on physician behavior, such as differences in hospitalization rates among patients treated in prepaid group practices and in fee-for-service practice and differences in the practices of physicians who do or do not own radiological equipment. He also discusses noneconomic reasons for variations in physician behavior, such as gray areas in which clear criteria do not exist to guide clinical decisions. He concludes that the different views of economists and physicians can be explained by differences in training and approaches to decisions and clinical practice and suggests that changes in the medical care market are bringing physicians closer to the economist's way of thinking.

Robert M. Veatch sheds light on the ethical issues that may be at stake in the emergence of for-profit enterprise in medical care by examining the history of medical codes of ethics. The codes have long exhibited concern about the commercialization of medicine and the possible subordination of physicians to lay control. Although the spread of for-profit health care companies may raise both sets of concerns,

Veatch sees medical codes as evolving toward greater compatibility with these developments. Veatch also examines more fundamental philosophical principles underlying the ethics of medicine and of commerce and finds that some significant areas of tension continue to exist.

One of the concerns about the involvement of physicians in for-profit enterprises, particularly when they are owners or share in profits, is that the physician's interest may conflict with the patient's interest. Frances H. Miller's paper analyzes how the law defines and views conflict of interest. She also examines the legal basis of the frequently expressed assertion that the physician has a fiduciary responsibility for the patient. Her analysis suggests that as physicians become more like businessmen they move further from the fiduciary role and possibly create legal situations that will deserve attention. Much of her analysis concerns the elements of the doctor-patient relationship that have led to the emergence of the view of the physician as occupying a position of trust. In general, these are not elements that are readily subject to change.

Conclusion

Although knowledgeable observers agree that the growth of the for-profit sector is a development of major significance, there is as yet little agreement and few facts about the meaning and implications of that growth. Does the development of for-profit medical care represent a change in the goals pursued by medical professionals and institutions, or is it only a change in the methods by which the traditional goals of service are pursued? Does the growth in for-profit health care represent a decline in the ideals that morally anchored a powerful profession and facilitated necessary patient trust, or does it embody a more honest acknowledgment of realities that have always been present? Or is it a neutral development?

Understanding the meaning and implications of a rapidly developing social change is never easy, particularly when that change, like the emergence of the for-profit health care sector, is taking place in an environment that is itself rapidly changing. Efforts are under way to change methods of paying for care in hopes of gaining better control over health care costs, which are exceeding general rates of inflation and consuming ever larger portions of the nation's wealth. Debate continues about the proper role of government in the health care system, although all levels of government are seeking to reduce their own expenditures for medical care, attempting both to cut costs and to shift costs elsewhere. Great uncertainty is expressed about how projected future capital requirements in health care will bo mot. New technologies that provide an opportunity for profit, which in some cases may encourage a more entrepreneurial orientation among physicians, continue to emerge from biomedical science. Coalitions of purchasers of care are organizing to exert pressures for controlling costs. Health policy is increasingly influenced by the belief in the benefits of greater competition among insurers and providers of health services and greater price sensitivity on the part of patients. The rapidly growing supply of physicians becomes a spur to more competition in health care. Activities of the organized medical professions are increasingly being challenged as restrictive of competition.

One of the most interesting aspects of the emergence of the for-profit sector is that, in this era of heavy government involvement in the financing and regulation of health care, no government program or policy set out to create a for-profit sector. Nevertheless, various governmental decisions have helped create an environment in which for-profit health care organizations have been able to compete very successfully. The public policy questions in the 1980s will revolve around the continuation of that environment.

Clearly, how best to provide and finance health services has assumed an important place on the public agenda. The future of those services will be shaped not only by impersonal economic and demographic forces but also by government policies. Some policies will be aimed specifically at the health care system—for example, on Medicare reimbursement for services or capital costs or on the process of gaining approval to build new health facilities—while others may not be intended primarily as *health* policy—for example, accelerated depreciation allowances intended to stimulate the U.S. economy and that were very helpful to the hospital companies. Ideally, future government actions will be based on an understanding of the meaning of the success of for-profit health care organizations and of the changes that are occurring in the medical profession and in medical institutions. It is our hope that these papers, and the subsequent Institute of Medicine study, will contribute to that understanding.

References and Notes

1. Arnold S. Relman, "The New Medical-Industrial Complex," *The New England Journal of Medicine* 303 (October 23, 1980), pp. 963-970.

2. Figures based on data from the Federation of American Hospitals in their directories for 1982 and 1983 and from the 1982 edition of *Hospital Statistics*, published by the American Hospital Association. In 1982 investor-owned hospitals comprised approximately 15 percent of U.S. hospitals. Of the 1,045 hospitals that made up this 15 percent, almost two-thirds (668) were owned by "management companies"—corporations that own several (by convention, at least three) hospitals. Some of these companies also manage hospitals under contract. The growth in the number of hospitals owned by management companies has been substantial, particularly in light of a slight decline in both the number of hospitals in the United States and in the investor-owned sector, as shown below:

Year	Total U.S. Hospitals	Community Hospitals	Independently Owned Proprietary Hospitals	Investor-Owned Chain Hospitals
1977	7,099	5,881	584	420
1981	6,933	5,813	not available	586
1982	not available	not available	377	668

Between 1977 and 1981 there was a 2 percent decline in the total number of hospitals, a 1 percent decline in the number of community hospitals, and a 40 percent expansion of management-company ownership, followed by another year of substantial growth (14 percent) in 1982. Clearly, management-company ownership of hospitals is growing in importance, accounting for 6 percent of all U.S. hospitals in 1977 and almost 10 percent in 1982.

The impact of management-company ownership is not equally distributed among states. In 1982, 38 percent of management-company-owned hospitals were in 2 states, California and Texas, while 10 states contained no management-company-owned hospitals.

Similarly, ownership is unevenly distributed among the management companies with one corporation, Hospital Corporation of America, owning 30 percent (202) of the nation's stock of hospitals owned by mangement corporations. Sixty-nine percent of management corporations' hospital ownership is concentrated in 17 percent (6) of the management companies.

3. *1982 Directory: Investor-Owned Hospitals and Hospital Management Companies* (Little Rock, Ark.: Federation of American Hospitals, 1981), p. 9.

4. Robert M. Cunningham, Jr., *The Healing Mission and the Business Ethic* (Chicago: Pluribus Press, 1982), p. 1.

5. National Center for Health Statistics, *The National Nursing Home Survey: 1977 Summary for the United States* (Hyattsville, Md.: Public Health Service, 1979), p. 9.

6. Relman, op. cit.

7. This estimate comes from Gary Stevenson, executive director of the National Association of Urgent Care Centers, and is quoted in Emily Friedman, "Slicing the Pie Thinner," *Hospitals* 56 (October 6, 1982), p. 64.

8. See the paper by Horty and Mulholland in this volume for more discussion about corporate restructuring of hospitals.

9. Paul Starr, *The Social Transformation of American Medicine* (New York: Basic Books, 1983), p. 23.

10. Bernard Barber, *The Logic and Limits of Trust* (New Brunswick, N.J.: Rutgers University Press, in press). The following discussion of trust is based on Barber's analysis.

11. Ibid.

12. William J. Goode, "Encroachment, Charlatanism, and the Emerging Profession: Psychology, Medicine, and Sociology," *American Sociological Review* 25:6 (1960), pp. 902-914.

13. *Principles of Medical Ethics of the American Medical Association.* This language was adopted in 1912 and remained in the "Principles" until the 1957 revision.

14. George Ritzer, *Working: Conflict and Change*, 2d ed. (Englewood Cliffs, N.J.: Prentice-Hall, 1977), p. 51. In this quotation, Ritzer refers to Eliot Freidson's influential critique of earlier sociological analyses of professionalism in *The Profession of Medicine* (New York: Dodd, Mead, 1970) and quotes from Paul Halmos, *Professionalization and Social Change: The Sociological Review Monograph* (Keele: University of Keele, 1973), p. 6.

15. See David Rosner, *A Once Charitable Enterprise: Hospitals and Health Care in Brooklyn and New York, 1885-1915* (Cambridge: Cambridge University Press, 1982); Morris J. Vogel, *The Invention of the Modern Hospital: Boston 1870-1930* (Chicago: University of Chicago Press, 1980); Paul Starr, *The Social Transformation of American Medicine* (New York: Basic Books, 1983); Rosemary Stevens, " 'A Poor Sort of Memory': Voluntary Hospitals and Government Before the Depression," *Milbank Memorial Fund Quarterly* 60 (Fall 1982), pp. 551-584.

16. Sister John Gabriel, "The Hospital and the Changing Social Order," *in* Arthur C. Bachmeyer and Gerhard Hartman, eds. *The Hospital in Modern Society* (New York: Commonwealth Fund, 1943), p. 19.

17. Jeff Goldsmith, *Can Hospitals Survive? The New Competitive Health Care Market* (Homewood, Ill.: Dow Jones-Irwin, 1982), pp. 178-180.

18. Victor R. Fuchs, "The Battle for Control of Health Care," *Health Affairs* 1 (Summer 1982), pp. 5-13; Friedman, op. cit., p. 62.

19. Robert C. Clark, "Does the Non-Profit Form Fit the Hospital Industry?" *Harvard Law Review* 93 (May 1980), pp. 1416-1489.

20. Relman, op. cit.

21. Goldsmith, op. cit.

22. See, for example, Lewin and Associates, *Studies in the Comparative Performance of Investor-Owned and Not-For-Profit Hospitals*, four volumes, Washington, D.C., Lewin and Associates, 1981.

Legal Differences Between Investor-Owned and Nonprofit Health Care Institutions

John F. Horty and Daniel M. Mulholland III

In recent years there has been a substantial increase in the number of investor-owned enterprises in the health care field, particularly hospitals.[1] This development has challenged some of the prevailing concepts and traditions of the field and of the professions engaged in it, particularly physicians. An increase in investor-owned enterprises in health care may have a number of political, economic, and social implications for the nation in general and the field in particular, but these implications cannot be adequately evaluated without an understanding of the basic legal differences between investor-owned and nonprofit health care institutions. This paper will examine these legal differences with respect to organization, finances, and miscellaneous factors.

Organizational Differences

With few exceptions, both investor-owned and nonprofit hospitals are organized as corporations. A handful of investor-owned hospitals may still be set up as general or limited partnerships (mostly those owned by a few physicians), and a few nonprofit hospitals may be organized as unincorporated associations, but the corporate form is so overwhelmingly prevalent in the field that this paper will address only the legal issues arising out of the use of the corporate form.

17

Investor-Owned Hospitals

Investor-owned hospitals are generally operated as either a separate proprietary "business" corporation or as subsidiaries of multihospital systems.[2] Even among the hospitals that are subsidiaries of holding company chains, however, many individual hospitals are separate corporations and responsible to a certain degree for their own affairs, subject to the ultimate control of the holding company. Thus, the discussion that follows is equally applicable to freestanding investor-owned hospitals and those integrated into hospital chains. It should be noted that while a substantial majority of investor-owned hospitals are freestanding the vast majority of investor-owned beds are owned by chains. In short, the chain investor-owned hospitals are considerably larger than the freestanding hospitals in the number of beds and thus in operating expenses.

All investor-owned corporations, regardless of whether they operate hospitals, are governed by the business corporation laws of the state in which they are incorporated. They must also register with other states in which they do business. Because of the relatively unobtrusive provisions of the business corporation laws of some states, e.g., Delaware, with respect to internal corporate operations, many corporations doing business in more than one state are incorporated under the laws of a state other than where they conduct the bulk of their business.[3] Corporations that only do business within one state, however, are more often than not incorporated only under that state's business corporation law.

There are certain basic attributes shared by all business corporations. All business corporations are ultimately governed by their shareholders, i.e., individuals or corporations who possess a proprietary interest in the assets and income of the corporation that is signified by the ownership of stock. The shareholders, as owners of the corporation, elect a board of directors, which is responsible for the conduct of the corporation.

The board of directors in turn employs various individuals who are responsible for the day-to-day operations of the corporation. These individuals are referred to as officers or agents of the corporation. In most cases, at least with respect to investor-owned companies, the officers of the corporation also are members of the board of directors. This is most frequently true of the chief executive officer of the corporation. Beyond this, it is difficult to identify any other general patterns of organization because the titles, functions, and relationships of the various elements of corporations differ from state to state as well as from corporation to corporation.

The purpose of most state corporate laws is to protect the rights of the shareholders in relation to the corporation's board or management. These laws set forth rules governing corporate elections, require the board to render periodic financial statements to the shareholders, and provide mechanisms by which shareholders who dissent from certain actions taken by the corporation can receive compensation for their shares in lieu of continuing their association with the corporation. There are few, if any, restrictions on the kinds of business that can be conducted by business corporations, aside from general prohibitions against conducting criminal activities. Thus, the stated-purpose clause of many investor-owned companies, including hospitals, generally permits the corporation to engage in "any lawful activities permitted to be conducted by corporations" in the particular state. This allows easy diversification of investor-owned corporations into both related and unrelated business.

The general and specific purposes of the corporation are outlined in the articles of incorporation or charter, the document filed with the state to obtain the state's recognition of the corporation's existence as a separate legal entity. More detailed rules governing the organization and operation of the corporation can be found in the bylaws of the corporation. Although state laws generally require that certain minimal information be included in the articles of incorporation, the corporation is usually free to fashion its bylaws in whatever way it sees fit.

In the case of hospitals, however, there are a number of additional regulatory and accreditation requirements pertaining to the content of the corporate bylaws that ultimately affect their organization, whether investor-owned or nonprofit. These include regulations promulgated by state departments of health or whatever state agency governs the conduct of hospitals. Such regulations traditionally dealt with "bricks and mortar" issues, such as safety standards and other public health concerns, but more recently they have begun to deal with the internal management of the hospital and to prescribe certain organizational requirements and restrictions. Likewise, the Joint Commission on Accreditation of Hospitals and the American Osteopathic Association, which together accredit almost all hospitals in the United States, have extensive standards pertaining to the internal organization and operation of the hospital board and management.[4] Thus, both investor-owned and nonprofit hospitals are not as free to fashion some portions of their bylaws as other corporations may be.

In addition to general regulations under state corporate statutes, business corporations that make their shares available for purchase by the public are subject to federal regulation under the federal securities laws, such as the Securities Act of 1933[5] and the Securities Exchange Act of 1934.[6] Corporations whose shares are available only to a limited number of shareholders and are not offered to the public are not subject to this regulation.

One of the major advantages of the chain holding company model for operating hospitals is that removing central management of the corporation from the local sites of the hospital allows major fiscal and operating decisions to be made free of local pressure, either from the community or from physicians. Thus, the local hospital is more likely to conform to the corporate fiscal plan with greater efficiency. In effect, local management has less discretion and is less likely to be manipulated by local community or physician interests through the board, because management is effectively employed and evaluated by the holding company. These are significant differences between the legal operation of the chain investor-owned hospital and the locally owned and operated nonprofit hospital.

Nonprofit Hospitals

The majority of hospitals (which represents the majority of hospital beds) are organized and operated as nonprofit corporations. They are subject to the nonprofit corporation laws of the states in which they are incorporated. Compared with business corporation laws, nonprofit corporation laws are far more varied through the country. Some general observations can nevertheless be made. There are two basic types of nonprofit corporations: membership and nonmembership.[7]

A membership corporation is more closely analogous to the investor-owned corporation in terms of its organization. A body of individuals known as the members is given the authority to elect a board of directors (or trustees as they are frequently called). In the case of a hospital the members may include individuals from the local community, representatives of a religious group affiliated with the hospital, physicians on the medical staff, or even other corporations. The board is responsible for the conduct of the corporation. The board in turn employs officers and agents to run the day-to-day affairs of the corporation. These individuals are known as either management or administration of the corporation.

The very use of the term *administration* instead of the generic corporate term *management* denotes the tradition in the nonprofit hospital corporation of giving the administrator—the individual who is the equivalent of the chief executive officer in a business corporation—less authority than his business counterpart. This tradition is changing, and the nonprofit manager now has greater authority, in part as a result of the growth of chain investor-owned hospitals.

State nonprofit corporation laws usually grant some degree of protection to the rights of members with respect to actions taken by the board or corporate management, e.g., prohibiting the board from unilaterally adopting any bylaws, amendments, or fundamental corporate changes that would affect the rights of the members[8] or requiring that the books and records of the corporation be open for inspection by the members.[9]

In most states, however, nonprofit corporations do not have to be organized as membership organizations, and, even where they are, it is permissible to have the membership and the board of trustees composed of the same individuals.[10] Thus, nonprofit corporations can be governed by self-perpetuating boards answerable only to themselves (and to state law) with respect to the internal affairs of the corporation. Although it would seem that a board and management of a corporation without members would have a far freer hand than their investor-owned counterparts in operating the corporation, generally there is little practical difference. Shareholders in business corporations seldom care about or exercise their prerogatives to change or restrict managements, as long as profits continue at an expected rate.

Where members are present, the board and management may possess less freedom, depending on the environment in which the corporation finds itself. This is especially true in the health care field. For example, hospitals located in areas with a strong tradition of community involvement by means of membership in the corporation will often have boards and management that are reluctant to embark on aggressive new or nontraditional hospital ventures for fear of upsetting some elements of the community, particularly the physicians. In such a situation the hospital corporation can become almost as highly politicized as a unit of local government. Other hospitals have corporate memberships composed completely or partially of the physicians on its medical staff.[11] This places the board in the rather peculiar position of having to answer to the same group whose medical quality it is responsible for overseeing.[12]

Corporate membership bodies can also provide a vehicle for certain factions within the hospital to wrest control from boards or management that they are displeased with. In many instances, anyone can become a member of the corporation upon payment of token dues, often as little as $5.00 per year. Thus, a group that is interested or astute enough can gather a substantial following and attempt a coup.[13] Some states even provide for derivative suits by members.[14] Fortunately for boards and management, this threat is largely diminished by the usual inertia of the membership, and it can be further blunted by carefully crafted bylaws that provide for more stringent membership requirements or that allow the board to approve new members or remove current ones.[15]

The courts generally have protected the rights of boards and management in such situations. For instance, in one case where a segment of the corporate membership of a hospital, during a dispute with the board, attempted to call a meeting on their own to remove the current board and elect a new one, an Illinois court invalidated that action and ruled in favor of the existing board, emphasizing that the hospital's bylaws did not permit that action.[16] The court went on to rule that members of nonprofit corporations have no constitutional right to elect or remove board members because, unlike shareholders in business corporations, they possess no property interest in the corporation.

In hospitals, perhaps more than other nonprofit institutions, it is essential that the board and management retain real control of the hospital. This is so not only because the nature and size of the business demand tight entrepreneurial control but also because various regulatory and accreditation bodies, as well as the courts, have placed the responsibility for running the hospital squarely on the shoulders of the board. For example, the Joint Commission on Accreditation of Hospitals requires that each hospital have "an organized governing body . . . that has overall responsibility for the conduct of the hospital. . . ."[17] Likewise, the Conditions of Participation for the federal Medicare program require that each hospital receiving reimbursement from the program have "an effective governing body legally responsible for the conduct of the hospital as an institution."[18] Many state licensing regulations have similar statements.[19] While revocation of license or accreditation for these reasons is rare, the threat is there and is perceived as real.

Most compelling, however, is the increasing number of judicial decisions in recent years holding that a hospital board is responsible for the quality of medical and hospital care rendered in the institution, even by nonemployees,[20] as well as for the fiscal integrity of the corporation.[21] If a hospital board is to fulfill its responsibilities in this area, it must exercise the ultimate authority within the corporation. In light of these realities, corporate bylaws that dilute the authority of the board, in favor of corporate members who may not be concerned with profit or the dynamic future of the corporation, are a threat to the well-being of the institution.

In most multihospital systems (both investor-owned and nonprofit) the authority of the board of each individual hospital within the system is necessarily circumscribed to some degree by the reserved powers of the controlling entity of the system. Nevertheless, the individual hospital boards will still be held legally responsible for the conduct of their respective institutions. Thus, in order to avoid an increased potential for liability, enough discretionary power to deal with internal concerns, especially medical staff affairs and quality assurance, must be given to the individual boards.

There are, however, some multihospital systems (mostly investor-owned) in which the individual hospitals are not separately incorporated. Rather, one corporation with one board owns all the hospitals collectively. This kind of arrangement, while possessing some tax advantages, has some serious drawbacks. The single corporate board will be held legally responsible for the conduct of each individual hospital, even though it is not as close to the day-to-day operations of the hospital as a local board would be. Also, creditors and tort claimants who are awarded judgments against one of the hospitals in the system can satisfy those judgments by attaching the assets of some or all of the other hospitals. This generally would not be possible if each hospital were separately incorporated.

Another factor that creates an important organizational distinction between investor-owned and nonprofit hospitals are the strictures imposed on the purposes for which nonprofit corporations can be organized and operated. First of all, almost all nonprofit corporation statutes require that the corporation be for a limited number of purposes, generally charitable, scientific, educational, benevolent, religious, etc.[22] Second, and this is probably the most fundamental difference between investor-owned and nonprofit corporations, the income and assets of the nonprofit corporation are not permitted to inure to the benefit of any private individual.[23]

This does not mean the corporation's board and management must serve without pay. It simply means that no private individuals, including the board and members, can exercise "ownership rights" in the corporation's assets as shareholders would with respect to the assets of a business corporation.[24] Other provisions in nonprofit corporation statutes can require judicial supervision of the dissolution of nonprofit corporations.[25] These statutes effectively prevent a whole range of entrepreneurial partnership arrangements that could bring equity capital into the corporation and that are routinely open to investor-owned hospitals.

Despite the fact that nonprofit corporations are subject to this restraint against private inurement, nonprofit corporations are not appendages of state or local governments. They are private institutions created pursuant to a statute but with a separate legal existence of their own. Therefore, it is incorrect to characterize their assets or operations as "public" assets or operations. Although those assets or operations may be devoted to a generally public or charitable purpose, and private individuals are prohibited from "profiting" from them, they are owned by and are the responsibility of a private nonprofit corporation.

As previously implied, the restraint against private inurement has been said to be a primary source of operational differences between investor-owned and nonprofit health care institutions. Some observers have concluded that the absence of a profit motive in nonprofit corporations leads managers of such institutions to seek "prestige" among their peers in lieu of monetary rewards.[25] This may channel energies, for good or bad, into expanding the physical plant or adding sophisticated technological equipment, without the requirement of profitability. This may be good for the availability of health care to the community but may be a risk to the long-term financial viability of the corporation. It has also been asserted that the professional beneficiaries of nonprofit institutions (in the case of hospitals, the medical staff) often fill the vacuum left by an absence of shareholder proprietors and dictate policies of the institution.[27] This is especially true where the board or management fails to exercise proper leadership.

At least one study has concluded that nonprofit hospitals are less efficient than their investor-owned counterparts in the ratio of personnel to the occupancy rate.[28] Other studies support the conclusion that managers in investor-owned hospitals perform better than those in nonprofit institutions because of the latter's lack of proprietary incentives.[29] Current statistics seem to bear this out, although the data unfortunately are not controlled for the mix and severity of cases. In 1981 investor-owned institutions had a lower average length of stay (6.5 days to 7.8) and lower full-time equivalent personnel per 100 adjusted census (322 to 348) than nonprofit hospitals.[30] And, while average daily expenses were slightly higher in investor-owned hospitals than in nonprofits ($299.02 compared with $285.61), labor costs were significantly lower in investor-owned hospitals than in nonprofits ($140.32 to $164.01 per inpatient day).[31]

These figures, which are commonly viewed as indices of efficiency in the health care field, would seem to indicate a marked advantage associated with the investor-owned form of organization. However, they must be viewed in light of the fact that many investor-owned institutions tend to have a higher proportion of "paying" patients as opposed to those whose bills are paid by third-party programs, such as Medicare, that reimburse at or below actual costs and that nonprofit hospitals are more likely to be engaged in costly teaching or training programs—programs whose costs center in the nonprofit field but whose benefits accrue to all.

Some investor-owned hospitals (as well as some nonprofits) have chosen not to participate in Medicare or accept charity patients at all or to set quotas (stated or unstated) on the number of such patients who will be treated. This had led to charges that some investor-owned hospitals have been "dumping" Medicare, Medicaid, and charity patients on their nonprofit neighbors, especially in areas such as southern Florida.[32] A larger percentage of Medicare patients, who because of age or type of illness, generally stay in a hospital longer and require more intensive nursing care, could explain, at least in part, the difference in "efficiency" figures between investor-owned and nonprofit hospitals. Thus, the meaning and explanation of reported differences between different types of hospitals is not clear, and more empirical research is warranted.

Where dumping of Medicare, Medicaid, or charity patients has allegedly taken place, the medical staffs of the nonprofit and investor-owned hospitals involved often consist of virtually the same physicians. This means that for one reason or another, the physicians have made a conscious decision to treat one segment of their patients in one hospital and others in another. Where the physicians own a proprietary interest in the investor-owned hospital, the reason behind their decision to admit only paying patients there is rather obvious. However, where the hospitals are all nonprofit, or where an investor-owned hospital chain is involved, the physician's actions may be dictated by policies adopted by the hospitals or by the expressed feeling of one of the hospitals that it has a "duty" to receive and care for all patients regardless of their ability to pay. Once again, too little empirical data are available to make a definitive analysis of the subject, but clear anecdotal examples exist.

To summarize, there are a number of significant differences in the way the law treats investor-owned and nonprofit hospitals with respect to their organization. While there also seem to be some statistical differences in the efficiency with which the two types of hospitals conduct their operations that favor the investor-owned form, it is not clear that these differences can be causally linked to the legal differences between the two forms except where the corporate decision making can be more "objective" when removed physically and organizationally from the local scene.

Financial Differences

Another set of possible determinants of different patterns of behavior between for-profit and nonprofit hospitals are the legal incentives and disincentives affecting their financial affairs. These factors, which include tax exemptions, reimbursement mechanisms, available sources of equity capital, and restrictions on certain transactions, are often the guiding force behind the major decisions made by health care institutions.

Tax Exemptions

The most significant factor affecting the financial affairs of nonprofit hospitals is the availability of an exemption from federal income tax under Section 501(c)(3) of the Internal Revenue Code. This exemption gives nonprofits an advantage by allowing them to devote more of their gross revenues to internal operations and expansion of the same. It also frees them from the necessity of basing decisions on tax implications, except where possible unrelated business taxable income may be involved.[33]

Even when the actual amount of tax would not be great (as is more and more the case with declining revenues and tax rates), an exemption under Section 501(c)(3) is important for other reasons. For one thing, it is a prerequisite to obtaining an exemption from federal Social Security taxes,[34] which can result in tremendous savings for hospitals because they tend to be labor-intensive operations. Also, it provides access to sources of support that otherwise would not be available, i.e., tax-deductible donations[35] and tax-exempt bond financing.[36]

Almost as valuable as federal tax exemptions are exemptions from state taxation. Traditionally, the most important of these are property tax exemptions, which are usually available to nonprofit corporations organized for charitable purposes in general or for hospitals in particular. Recently, however, tax exemptions for hospitals in a few states have been successfully attacked by local taxing authorities using the theory that because hospitals receive reimbursement from third parties for almost all the care they provide they are no longer "charitable" operations.[37] Other state tax provisions of significance to nonprofit hospitals include exemptions from state sales taxes (for hospital purchases) and corporate income taxes.

Reimbursement Factors

Until recently, conventional wisdom held that nonprofit hospitals had a decided financial advantage over their investor-owned counterparts because of their tax exemptions. Lately though, it has been observed that certain factors involved in third-party reimbursement schemes, particularly Medicare, favor investor-owned hospitals and may counterbalance or even outweigh the tax advantages of nonprofits.[38]

As a result of repeated budget cuts, the Medicare program now reimburses all hospitals at less than their actual costs for treating Medicare patients. This is largely due to the reimbursement limits imposed on routine inpatient costs by Section 223 of the Medicare amendments of 1972 and the regulations thereunder.[39] If these limits are extended to ancillary services, this shortfall will be exacerbated. Faced with inadequate reimbursement from major third-party payers, hospitals are forced to make up the difference from paying patients or commercial insurance carriers. Many nonprofit hospitals are reluctant or unable to do this, either because of their historical mission to serve the poor, their location in predominantly poor or aging neighborhoods, or legal requirements that they render a certain percentage of their services without compensation in return for having received federal construction funds under the Hill-Burton Act.[40]

Investor-owned hospitals, on the other hand, are in most cases under no obligation to provide charity care and are more likely to accept only patients for which they will be reimbursed in full. Furthermore, investor-owned hospitals are entitled to third-party payments that nonprofits are not. The most prominent of these is reimbursement for a reasonable "return on equity" in addition to costs under the Medicare program.[41] This return on equity recently has been paid at rates upward of 22 percent of net equity.[42] Investor-owned hospitals are therefore guaranteed a "profit" that is denied nonprofit hospitals. In addition, many federal and state taxes are allowable costs under the Medicare program,[43] so the tax advantage of the tax-exempt nonprofit hospital is further reduced.

Sources of Capital

At first glance, nonprofit hospitals would seem to have an advantage in attracting new capital because of the tax deductibility of contributions to them and the availability of tax-exempt bonds. Indeed, this latter category of financing has become almost crucial to the survival of the nonprofit side of the industry. As of 1981 it is estimated that over $5 billion worth of tax-exempt hospital bonds have been issued.[44] These bonds are the primary source of funding for hospital construction, financing 49.3 percent of such activity in 1978, compared with 6.2 percent from philanthropy and 8.6 percent from government funds.[45] The tax-exempt feature enables nonprofit hospitals to issue bonds with higher ratings and lower interest rates than would otherwise be possible, thereby increasing their marketability and decreasing expenses.[46] The concept of tax-exempt bonds is under increasing federal government scrutiny, and the future is uncertain.

Private charitable contributions to nonprofit hospitals have decreased in importance over the years, mostly as a result of the advent of Medicare and the consequent shifts of donor interest to other fields. This trend probably will accelerate, as recent tax code changes reduce the incentive for taxpayers to contribute to charities. The Economic Recovery Tax Act of 1981[47] reduced the maximum rates of both federal income and estate taxes, which could work to discourage some larger donors from contributing, because the value of the deduction they would receive is less. Also, the general economic downturn during 1982 can be expected to diminish charitable giving.

At the same time, investor-owned hospitals are not as disadvantaged by the lack of access to the tax-exempt bond market as one might expect. In the first place, tax-exempt financing is available under limited circumstances to investor-owned hospitals under the so-called small issue exemption.[48] Moreover, third-party payers, including Medicare, usually reimburse hospitals for their borrowing costs.[49] Some observers have even claimed this fact renders normal borrowing more beneficial to the hospital than tax-exempt borrowing since the savings realized from the tax exemption are passed on to the third-party payers.[50]

Investor-owned hospitals also can resort to the most traditional method of raising capital—issuing stock—which is unavailable to nonprofit hospitals in most states.[51] However, some of the larger investor-owned chains have reduced their reliance on this method of financing in recent months, opting instead for bonds, debentures, and short-term notes, because of a downward trend in their stock prices caused by government indecision over reimbursement.[52] This provides further support for the theory that debt financing is not as unattractive to investor-owned hospitals as was previously thought.

Restrictions on Transfers of Property

Many state laws governing nonprofit corporations prohibit the transfer of funds restricted for specific charitable purposes without judicial approval.[53] For example, if a nonprofit hospital solicited and received donations that were earmarked by their terms for the construction of a new surgical suite and some of those funds were left over after the suite was constructed, the hospital would have to obtain a court order allowing it to use the excess funds for other purposes. These restrictions, which find their origins in the law of charitable trusts, can be burdensome in the sophisticated business environment in which hospitals find themselves. They could also give rise to significant problems when hospitals needing to convert dormant assets, such as real estate, into ready cash face restrictions that were attached to the use of the asset when it was donated.

Some states have laws that permit the state attorney general to institute investigation and enforcement actions concerning alleged misuse of charitable gifts by nonprofit corporations, presumably even where there are no explicit restrictions imposed by the donor.[54] Others require membership approval before transfers of property can be made.[55] Such statutes have the potential of hindering the financial conduct of nonprofit corporations, although in practice they may not be strictly enforced.[56] Moreover, because the majority of nonprofit hospitals are small, independent, local corporations, they lack the ability of the investor-owned chains to transfer assets between hospital units as needed and to guarantee large loans and bond issues, very important fiscal tools in today's financial market.

It is impossible to generalize whether the nonprofit or the investor-owned form is most advantageous for hospitals with respect to their financial transactions. While it is true that many advantages historically possessed by nonprofit institutions have eroded over the years, the tax exemptions that are usually available to nonprofits still provide a powerful incentive for them to retain that status. Only a careful analysis on an institution-specific basis can determine which form best suits a hospital from a financial point of view in light of current or forecast legislative or regulatory realities. In the end, given inadequate reimbursement for care of the elderly and poor, the major fiscal disadvantage of the nonprofit hospital may be community, state, and federal expectations of the role of such hospitals.

Other Legal Differences

Another set of legal differences between investor-owned and nonprofit hospitals are laws requiring a greater degree of public "accountability" from nonprofit hospital governing boards. West Virginia, for instance, has enacted a law requiring nonprofit hospital board meetings to be open to the public,[57] much the same as board meetings of governmentally owned and operated institutions must be in a number of states. Investor-owned hospitals are excluded from this requirement, presumably to protect their business data and plans from competitors, which in most areas are nonprofit hospitals. In contrast, Pennsylvania requires all hospitals to provide "some opportunity for the general public to attend meetings of the governing body on occasion. . . ."[58] The problem with such open-meeting requirements is not that board meetings will be overwhelmed by a flood of spectators; most people couldn't care less what goes on with a hospital board. Rather, the presence of reporters or possibly competitors—who are more likely to attend than the general public—will hamper the board if it has to discuss sensitive or confidential matters, such as financing options, legal positions, or medical staff credentialing.

Nonprofit hospitals previously enjoyed fairly broad exemptions from certain federal regulatory schemes, but these have been crumbling as of late. For example, in 1974 most federal labor laws, including the National Labor Relations Act and the wage and hour laws, were made applicable to nonprofit hospitals. Previously, only proprietary hospitals had been covered. Likewise, many federal antitrust laws have only recently been applied to nonprofit hospitals.

In *Hospital Building Company* v. *Trustees of Rex Hospital*,[59] the Supreme Court ruled for the first time that the activities of a nonprofit hospital had enough impact on interstate commerce to bring the hospital under the jurisdiction of the Sherman Act.[60] In another case that same year,[61] the Court ruled that the Robinson-Patman Act, which forbids price discrimination in favor of large buyers over smaller ones, applied to nonprofit hospitals under certain circumstances despite a provision of the act that exempted sales to charitable institutions.[62]

About the only antitrust law that has not been applied to nonprofit hospitals is the Federal Trade Commission Act, which by its terms applies only to investor-owned institutions.[63] This has not prevented the FTC from successfully attacking certain actions of health-related trade groups, such as the American Medical Association,[64] or from aggressively challenging certain acquisitions made by investor-owned hospital chains.[65]

Conclusion

As this paper has shown, there are a number of differences in the way the law treats investor-owned and nonprofit hospitals. While many of these differences can reasonably be expected to influence the operations of hospitals, as well as their finances, it is impossible to identify any general trends along these lines in the absence of empirical studies conducted on a large-scale, institution-specific basis.

The distinction between nonprofit and investor-owned hospitals has been blurred by the recent move toward corporate restructuring by many nonprofit hospitals. The usual corporate restructuring plan has a single-hospital corporation evolve into a holding company with a number of subsidiaries, one of which is the hospital. The other subsidiaries may be investor-owned or nonprofit, depending on the activity to be conducted. However, even in this area, nonprofit hospitals lag behind those that are investor-owned. Because business corporations are owned by shareholders, it is relatively easy to merge them into multicorporate systems under the umbrella of a holding company that owns all of their stock. Moreover, as stated earlier, it is relatively easy to transfer assets between parent and subsidiary business corporations.

Nonprofit corporations, however, are not technically owned by anyone, so the holding company idea is somewhat foreign to them. Only quite recently have nonprofit hospitals ventured into the restructuring arena and even then with a good deal of reluctance. One fairly popular method of nonprofit restructuring—creating a nonprofit holding company and making it the sole member of the hospital corporation—will not work in those states discussed earlier that prohibit the transfer of nonprofit corporate income to corporate members. Thus, other, more unfamiliar methods must be employed. Nonprofits also have been far slower than investor-owned companies to establish hospital chains for the same reason.

Although the original impetus for restructuring was a desire to enhance reimbursement by spinning off nonreimbursible activities into sister corporations, many hospitals have begun to realize that even greater benefits can be obtained by restructuring to positioning themselves for competition with other hospitals, especially those affiliated with investor-owned chains or other multihospital systems.

Increased competition may ultimately break down many of the existing differences between investor-owned and nonprofit hospitals. If third-party reimbursement levels continue to decline, or if legislation mandating price competition between providers, such as the National Healthcare Reform Act of 1981,[66] is adopted, hospitals of all stripes will be forced to act like business corporations if they are to survive. Under such circumstances, existing laws and regulations restricting the activities of nonprofit hospitals will become anachronisms, destined to fall in the wake of new realities.

32   JOHN F. HORTY and DANIEL M. MULHOLLAND III

References and Notes

1. As of 1981 there were 6,933 hospitals in the United States. Of this number, 5,813 were described by the American Hospital Association as community hospitals, i.e., hospitals not owned by the federal government or devoted solely to treating pyschiatric or respiratory problems. Of the community hospitals, 3,340 were owned by nonprofit organizations, 1,744 by state or local governmental units, and 729 by investor-owned companies. Interestingly, the number of investor-owned hospitals has actually decreased in recent years, as well as over the long term, but the number of beds owned or managed by them has increased dramatically, from approximately 57,000 in 1972 to 88,000 in 1981. By the same token, the number of nonprofit beds only increased from 617,000 to 706,000 during the same period, and state and local government beds increased from 205,000 to 210,000. (Source: American Hospital Association, *Hospital Statistics*, 1982 edition, Table 1, pp. 5-7.)

Using a different definition and different data collection methods, the Federation of American Hospitals—the trade association of the investor-owned hospitals—reported that in 1981 there were 1,376 investor-owned hospitals with 159,314 beds. Of these, 942 hospitals (with 121,741 beds) were owned by the investor-owned management companies. (Source: *1982 Directory: Investor-Owned Hospitals and Hospital Management Companies* (Little Rock, Ark.: Federation of American Hospitals, 1982), p. 9.)

2. A recent survey of 172 multihospital systems revealed that 107,765 acute care hospital beds in the United States are controlled by investor-owned chains, 170,866 by nonprofit multihospital systems, and 18,453 by governmental systems. The Hospital Corporation of America alone controlled 48,484 beds. See Donald E. L. Johnson and Linda Punch, "Multihospital Systems Survey," *Modern Healthcare* 12 (May 1982), pp. 67-130.

3. Del. Code Ann. Tit. 8; see H. Henn *Corporations* (2d ed.) Sec. 93, p. 138, *et seq.*

4. See, JCAH, *Accreditation Manual for Hospitals*, 1982 ed.; AOA *Requirements and Interpretative Guide for Accredited Hospitals*, 1982.

5. 15 U.S.C. Sec. 77.

6. 15 U.S.C. Sec. 78.

7. These have also been referred to as "mutual" and "entrepreneurial" nonprofits, respectively. See Henry B. Hansmann, "The Role of Nonprofit Enterprise," *Yale Law Journal* 89 (April 1980), pp. 835-901.

8. 15 Pa. C.S.A. Sec. 7504.

9. Ohio Rev. Code Sec. 1702.15; Wis. Stat. Ann. Sec. 181.27.

10. See Fla. Stat. Ann. Sec. 617.025.

11. This is especially true for many osteopathic hospitals founded by osteopathic physicians during the 1940s and 1950s, when allopathic institutions refused to grant them privileges. Such discrimination recently has been ruled invalid by the courts—see, e.g., *Greisman* v. *Newcomb Hospital*, 192 A.2d 817 (N.J. 1963) and *Don* v. *Okmulgee Memorial Hospital*, 443 F.2d 234 (10th Cir. 1971)—but its legacy, the osteopathic hospital, still exists.

12. It is universally acknowledged that the governing board of a hospital is responsible for the overall conduct of the hospital, including the medical staff. See, e.g., *Khan* v. *Suburban Community Hospital*, 340 N.E.2d 398 (Ohio 1976) and *Schulman* v. *Washington Hospital Center*, 222 F.Supp. 59 (D.C. 1963).

13. In one unreported instance this was attempted by the nurses at a hospital who persuaded enough of their relatives and friends to become corporate members and oust a group of trustees perceived as hostile to the nurses.

14. Wis. Stat. Ann. Sec. 181.295, N.Y. Not-For-Profit Corp. Law Sec. 631. See also *Atwell* v. *Bide-a-Wee Home Association*, 299 N.Y.S.2d 40 (Sup. Ct. 1969), which gave contributors who are *not* members of a nonprofit corporation the right to bring derivative actions.

15. Needless to say, the fact that nonprofit boards have the ability to control the corporation's membership has not met with approval in all quarters. See, generally, Jane L. Davis, "Membership Rights in Nonprofit Corporations: A Need for Increased Legal Rec-

ognition and Protection," *Vanderbilt Law Review* 29 (1976), p. 747; Robin Dimieri and Stephen Weiner, "The Public Interest and Governing Boards of Nonprofit Health Care Institutions," *Vanderbilt Law Review* 34 (May 1981), p. 1029.

16. *Harris* v. *Board of Directors of Community Hospital of Evanston*, 370 N.E.2d 1121 (Ill. App. 1977).

17. JCAH, *Accreditation Manual for Hospitals*, 1982 ed., p. 51.

18. 42 C.F.R. Sec. 405.1021.

19. E.g., 28 Pa. Code Sec. 103.1 (1982); Hospital Licensing Requirements, Illinois Department of Public Health, Sec. 2-1.1 (1981).

20. E.g., *Darling* v. *Charleston Community Hospital*, 211 N.E.2d 253 (Ill. 1965); *Johnson* v. *Misericordia Community Hospital*, 294 N.W.2d 501 (Wis. App. 1980); *aff'd* 301 N.W.2d (Wis. 1981).

21. *Stern* v. *Lucy Webb Hayes National Training School of Deaconesses and Missionaries*, 381 F.Supp. 1003 (D.D.C. 1974).

22. While some states permit nonprofits to be organized for "any lawful business"—see, e.g., New York Not-for-Profit Corporation Law Sec. 201—corporate purposes must be limited to charitable, educational, religious, or scientific pursuits to qualify for a federal tax exemption under Sec. 501(c)(3) of the Internal Revenue Code.

23. Howard Oleck, *Nonprofit Corporations, Organizations and Associations*, 3d ed. (Englewood Cliffs, N.J.: Prentice-Hall, 1979), p. 10. This prohibition against private inurement is also a prerequisite to an exemption under Sec. 501(c)(3) of the Internal Revenue Code.

24. Or as one observer put it: "The sources of equity capital retain no proprietary interest in it." Richard D. Wittrup, "Economic Behavior of Social Institutions," *Hospital Administration* (Winter 1975), pp. 8-16.

25. E.g., Pa. Const. Stat. Ann. Tit. 15 Sec. 7968(b).

26. Bruce C. Vladeck, "Why Nonprofits Go Broke," *Public Interest* 42:1 (1976), p. 86. See also Joseph P. Newhouse, "Toward a Theory of Nonprofit Institutions: An Economic Model of a Hospital," *American Economic Review* 60:1 (1970), p. 64.

27. Richard D. Wittrup, *supra* at 11.

28. William Rushing, "Differences in Profit and Nonprofit Organizations: A Study of Effectiveness and Efficiency in General Short Stay Hospitals," *Administrative Science Quarterly* 19 (1974), p. 474.

29. Kenneth W. Clarkson, "Some Implications of Property Rights in Hospital Management," *Journal of Law Economics* 15 (1972), p. 363; See, generally, Robert C. Clark, "Does the Nonprofit Form Fit the Hospital Industry?" *Harvard Law Review* 93 (1980), pp. 1417, 1460-1462.

30. American Hospital Association, *Hospital Statistics*, 1982 ed., Table 3, pp. 12-13.

31. Id. One possible explanation for the slightly higher overall expense figure is that many investor-owned hospitals, especially those in chains, are newer and therefore are still depreciating large capital expenditures.

32. With further cuts in Medicare funding an almost certain prospect, it can be expected that this trend will be exacerbated. See Richard L. Johnson, "The Resurgence of a Two Tier Health Care System," *Action-Kit Newsletter* (Pittsburgh: Action Kit for Health Law, August 1982). Linda K. Demkovich, "Urban Voluntary Hospitals Caught in Price Squeeze Face a Bleak Future," *National Journal* 15 (June 26, 1982), p. 1131.

33. Sec. 512-513, Internal Revenue Code.

34. Sec. 3121(b)(8)(B), Internal Revenue Code.

35. Sec. 170(b)(1)(A)(iii), Internal Revenue Code.

36. Secs. 103(b)(2)(A) and (3)(B), Internal Revenue Code.

37. See, *In re Appeal of Doctor's Hospital*, 414 A.2d 134 (Pa. Commw. 1980); *West Allegheny Hospital* v. *Board of Property Assessment*, No. 1171 C.D. 1980 (Pa. Commw. December 31, 1981). The latter case is currently on appeal to the Pennsylvania Supreme Court.

38. John S. Hoff and Kenneth I. Schaner, "Government Policies Force Nonprofits to Go For-Profit," *Modern Healthcare* 12 (June 1982), pp. 81-85.

39. 42 U.S.C. Sec. 1395x(v)(1); 42 C.F.R. Sec. 405.460.

40. 42 U.S.C. Sec. 291c(e)(2).

41. 42 C.F.R. Sec. 405.429.

42. Hoff and Schaner, *supra* n. 42 at 82.

43. Provider Reimbursement Manual Part I, Sec. 2122. Excluded are fines and penalties, income taxes, taxes associated with financing, sales taxes collected by the hospital, and taxes on property not used to provide covered services.

44. Taddey and Gayer, "Uses and Effects of Hospital Tax-Exempt Financing," *Healthcare Financial Management* 12 (July 1982), p. 10.

45. Id.

46. Id.

47. P.L. 97-34.

48. Sec. 103(b)(6), Internal Revenue Code. This exemption will be phased out by 1986 as a result of the Tax Equity and Fiscal Responsibility Act of 1982, P.L. 97-248 Sec. 214(c).

49. See, generally, 42 C.F.R. Sec. 405.419.

50. Hoff and Schaner, *supra* n. 41, at 82.

51. New York and Pennsylvania, however, permit nonprofit corporations to issue a form of security known as "subvention certificates," which closely resemble preferred stock to members or nonmembers, and to accept capital contributions from members. N.Y. Not-for-Profit Corp. Law Secs. 202(7) and (8), Secs. 504 and 505; Pa. Cons. Stat. Ann. Tit. 15 Secs. 7541 and 7542. These features have been criticized by some observers as making nonprofit corporations too "businesslike," see Oleck, *supra* n. 23 at 48-49, and there is no evidence that they have been widely used by hospitals in those states.

52. Esther F. Kuntz, "Chains Shy Away from Equity Financing," *Modern Healthcare* 12 (May 1982), p. 116.

53. E.g., Pa. Const. Stat. Ann. Tit. 15 Sec. 7549(b); W. Va. Code Secs. 35-2-1, 35-2-2.

54. Cal. Gov. Code Sec. 12580 *et seq.*; Ill. Rev. Stats. Ch. 14 Sec. 51 *et seq.*; N.Y. Est. Powers and Trusts Laws Sec. 8-1.4; Ohio Rev. Code Sec. 109.33.

55. Tex. Nonprofit Corp. Act, Art. 1396-2.13 requires the approval of the voting members where a quorum of at least one-tenth is present.

56. Oleck, *supra* n. 23, at 901-904.

57. W. Va. Code Sec. 16-5G-1.

58. 28 Pa. Code Sec. 103.3(10)(iii).

59. 425 U.S. 738 (1976).

60. 15 U.S.C. Sec. 1.

61. *Abbot Laboratories* v. *Portland Retail Druggist Association*, 425 U.S. 1 (1976).

62. 15 U.S.C. Sec. 13c.

63. 15. U.S.C. Sec. 44.

64. See *American Medical Association* v. *Federal Trade Commission*, 638 F.2d 443 (2d Cir. 1981); *aff'd*, 50 U.S.L.W. 4313 (March 23, 1982).

65. "Hospital Corporation Faced with Trust Suit by FTC," *Wall Street Journal* August 3, 1982, p. 6.

66. H.R. 850, introduced by Rep. Richard Gephardt (D-MO) and former Rep. David Stockman (R-MI), now Director of the Office of Management and Budget.

Wall Street and the For-Profit Hospital Management Companies

Richard B. Siegrist, Jr.

Ten years ago it would have been difficult to find a Wall Street analyst who seriously followed the for-profit hospital management companies,* much less one who would recommend that a client purchase the stock of any of these companies. Today the situation is drastically different. Approximately 25 security analysts spend half their time following the investor-owned hospital chains and would not hesitate to recommend the purchase of stock in these companies to almost any of their clients. In addition to these so-called sell side analysts, hundreds of portfolio managers, investment analysts, and retail stockbrokers keep in close touch with the performance of the for-profit hospital companies.

This paper will explore why the investment community's interest in the for-profit hospital companies has burgeoned and will address some basic questions about the hospital management industry:

1. Where does Wall Street obtain its information about the for-profit hospital companies? How does it use this information to evaluate them?

---

* Although conventionally referred to as "hospital management companies," it is these firms' *ownership* of hospitals that is of most relevance to this paper. However, the conventional "management" term will be used throughout.

2. How important is stock price to the management of the for-profit hospital chains?

3. Why have the hospital management companies been so successful?

4. What differences exist among the companies in this industry?

5. How are the hospital management companies able to acquire other hospitals and hospital chains? What difficulties do they face in doing so?

6. How are the companies able to turn distressed hospitals into profitable ones?

7. What is the future outlook for the hospital management industry?

This paper is based on conversations with about 10 Wall Street sell side analysts, supplemented with written reports prepared by the analysts, company annual reports, and information gained from research for earlier projects.[1] For most of the matters discussed here, there was a general consensus among the analysts, and the discussion is so presented. Instances where the analysts disagreed are noted.

The hospital management industry is dominated by five large companies: Hospital Corporation of America (HCA), Humana, American Medical International (AMI), National Medical Enterprises (NME), and Lifemark. Together they own approximately 6 percent of the acute care beds in the United States and represent about half of the beds owned by all for-profit hospitals.[2] Their growth in only the last five

TABLE 1 Size of the Five Largest Hospital Management Companies

	Net Revenue (millions)		Acute Care Beds Owned[a]	
	1981	1976	1981	1976
HCA	$2,064	$ 456	28,049	11,196
Humana	1,343	261	16,431	8,370
AMI	914	272	9,898	5,702
NME	892	116	4,717	2,068
Lifemark	273	71	3,725	1,573
TOTAL	$5,486	$1,186	62,820	28,909

[a]Includes international beds owned but excludes all beds managed under management contracts.

SOURCE: Company 1981 annual reports and 10K reports filed with the Securities and Exchange Commission.

years has been tremendous. Table 1 presents the net revenues and number of beds owned for these five companies in 1981 compared with 1976.

Analysts' Sources of Information

The investment community can be divided into four major groups of decision makers:[3]

1. Sell side analysts who specialize by industry and follow the companies in that industry very closely. Approximately 25 sell side analysts follow the for-profit hospital management companies. These analysts usually follow hospital supply and/or drug companies as well.
2. Buy side analysts or institutional investors. This group includes portfolio managers and security analysts for pension funds, banks, insurance companies, mutual funds, etc. There are approximately 10,000 such institutional investors.
3. Registered representatives or account executives at brokerage firms. There are about 35,000 retail stockbrokers.
4. Individual investors (i.e., the public).

The sell side analysts are a primary source of information and recommendations concerning the hospital management companies for the rest of the investment community. Because of the analysts' key role and their perspective on the industry, this paper focuses on their relationship with and evaluation of the hospital management companies.

The sell side analysts use a variety of written and oral sources of information in performing their analyses of investor-owned hospital chains. The most important written sources of information are publications from the companies themselves, industry periodicals, and government statistics. As publicly held corporations, the hospital management companies must prepare annual reports (reports to shareholders that contain audited financial statements and other financial and nonfinancial information); 10Ks (reports filed annually with the Securities and Exchange Commission (SEC), which contain audited financial statements and descriptions of company business and property); and 10Qs (interim quarterly reports filed with the SEC that contain unaudited financial information). Most companies supplement this required information with fact sheets, data books, and other publications that provide additional financial, operational, and strategic information.

Perhaps more valuable to the analysts than written sources of data are personal contacts, which enable analysts to obtain the most up-to-date information and to focus on topics about which they want more detailed information. The analysts obtain information orally from company officers, other industry analysts, health care experts, and federal and state government officials. Contact with legislators and their staffs in Washington has become even more critical in recent years, because of the increased scrutiny the hospital sector has been receiving and the expectation that the regulatory environment may change substantially.

The sell side analysts maintain close relationships with the for-profit hospital management companies that they follow. An analyst typically would be in contact with each of the major companies at least once a month. The contact person at a company is generally a high-level officer, such as the chief executive officer, vice-president of finance, or vice-president for investor relations. The fact that such high-level corporate officials personally deal with the analysts is a measure of their importance to the companies.

The analysts generally report that the hospital management industry is much more open and willing to provide information than many other industries. The analysts rate the companies very highly in providing useful written information and being accessible for questions. Although they perceive some slight differences among the five major companies in the quality of information and accessibility of management, the analysts believe that all of the major for-profit hospital management companies are very responsive to their needs. The openness of these companies may stem from the newness of their industry and their desire to increase investor recognition of the industry and interest in the companies' stocks. This openness appears to have contributed to the industry's success.

The sell side analysts as a group do not spend much time following the not-for-profit hospital chains. Aside from the fact that these systems do not sell stock, the analysts do not see them as a serious threat to the for-profit chains and thus not a group to be followed regularly. In addition, the analysts cite the dearth of information available from the not-for-profit systems and their general lack of accessibility, especially in comparison with the for-profit companies, as reasons why they do not pay much attention to the not-for-profit hospital systems.

Financial Analyses of Companies

The sell side analysts use a variety of different techniques in evaluating the hospital management companies: general industry evaluation, financial statement analysis, operational analysis, assessment of the quality of management, and stock price evaluation. The analysis of the hospital management companies can be different from the analysis of companies in other industries. Traditional rules of thumb (e.g., regarding debt/equity ratios) or financial relationships often do not apply to the hospital management industry.

An analysis of the overall situation of the hospital industry entails an examination of changing demographics, general economic conditions, business attitudes toward health care costs, and government regulation both on the national and state levels. This broad industry examination is supplemented with detailed financial statement analysis of the hospital management companies. Consistency and predictability are the key factors in analyses, according to the analysts.

The detailed examination of a company would include analysis of the balance sheet (with particular focus on financial leverage, i.e., degree of reliance on debt to finance total assets), the income statement (with emphasis on earnings growth, operating margin, and return on equity), and cash flow. An evaluation of operational considerations is another central part of the review. Facility location, the mix of sources of payers and rates paid for services, and case mix and intensity of services are important operational factors in an evaluation.

The analysts also place considerable emphasis on the quality of management. They look for management depth, ability to adapt quickly to change, an innovative outlook, and a well-planned strategy.

A final tool used by the analysts is stock price analysis. The analysts look to a stock's price/earnings ratio, price movement over time (technical analysis), dividend yield, and degree of institutional ownership in formulating recommendations as to whether the stock appears to be a good buy. The degree of institutional investment indicates the confidence that institutional investors have in the stock on the basis of their own assessments.

The Importance of Stock Prices to the Companies

The security analysts are not the only ones concerned about stock prices. Top officers of the hospital management companies place considerable emphasis on the price of their company's stock. There are several reasons for this concern. First, the stock price may be an important factor in making acquisitions. A high price in relation to earnings (i.e., a high price/earnings ratio) may permit a company to use its stock as a cheap source of capital to buy another hospital or a hospital chain. For instance, HCA was able to purchase Hospital Af-

filiates International (HAI), the second-largest hospital chain, by issuing $225 million of common stock for a third of the acquisition price,
representing a 12 percent increase in its shares for outstanding stock.
At the time, HCA shares were selling for 24 times 1980 earnings.[4] If
the multiple were lower due to a lower stock price, HCA would have
had to issue more shares, further diluting its equity, and may not
have been able to make the purchase.

Second, top officials of the companies own a significant number of
shares. Their individual wealth is thus directly affected by stock price.
A drop of several points could mean hundreds of thousands of dollars.
Table 2 below indicates the extent of management's stock ownership
in the five major companies.

Third, the top management at many of the companies receive stock
options and bonuses that are tied to the performance of the stock.
Finally, the desire of top management to retain the investment community's interest in the company magnifies its concern over the level
of the stock price.

Top management's interest in stock price can manifest itself in
several different ways, often varying by company. All the companies
are concerned about showing steady earnings per share growth because of the favorable impact this tends to have on price. The companies, however, differ somewhat in their time frame for stock price.
HCA appears more interested in short-term stock price than does
Humana, where management controls much more of the stock and
may have a longer-term orientation toward price.

A company's dividend policy also can affect its stock price. In general, the hospital management companies have low dividend payouts
in comparison with other industries. However, there are differences
in dividend policy within the hospital management industry. For ex-

TABLE 2 Percentage of Common Stock
Ownership by Top Management
(including directors), 1981

HCA	5
Humana	22
AMI	4
NME	9
Lifemark	4

SOURCE: Company prospectuses and proxy statements.

TABLE 3   Stock Price Trends Among the Hospital Management
Companies, 1977–1981

	Year-End Stock Price (after adjustment for general inflation)		Multiple of 1981 Price to 1976
	1981	1977	
HCA	$ 33.02	$ 13.12	2.5
Humana	31.50	4.88	6.5
AMI	24.83	7.00	3.6
NME	25.73	6.88	3.7
Lifemark	28.00	8.07	3.5
Dow Jones industrial average (unadjusted for inflation)	875.00	831.77	1.05

SOURCE: 1981 company annual reports.

ample, AMI had a much higher dividend payout at 27 percent of 1981
earnings than HCA at 15 percent of earnings.[5]

Finally, the willingness of management to dilute the equity of the
company by issuing more common stock varies considerably. Humana
is less willing than the other companies to issue common stock because
of management's reluctance to dilute its sizable interest (22 percent
ownership of the stock) in the company.

The hospital companies' stocks have performed phenomenally well
over the last decade. Table 3 shows the magnitude of the rise in stock
prices between 1977 and 1981 for the five major companies, after
adjustment for general inflation.

Reasons for Success of the Hospital Management Companies

The sell side analysts cite four primary reasons for the remarkable
success of the hospital management companies: access to capital, a
favorable environment, economies of scale, and quality of management.

The most commonly stated reason for success is the for-profit chains'
access to capital, especially in comparison with the nonprofit hospital
sector. The investor-owned firms can use a variety of financial instruments that are either not legally available to nonprofit hospitals
or require a strong financial position to qualify for. The most obvious
capital source that is available only to for-profit companies is equity,
i.e., the issuance of shares of stock. Although equity has played a role
in the growth of these companies, debt has been much more important.

The investor-owned companies have been able to use a variety of debt instruments, including domestic bank loans, Eurodollar financing, commercial paper, convertible debt, subordinated debentures, and industrial revenue bonds as well as traditional mortgage financing.

The effective use of debt financing or leverage has been central to the rapid growth of these companies. The hospital management industry is one of the most highly leveraged industries in the United States, with debt ranging from 60 to 85 percent of the capital structure of these companies, compared with the typical industrial company with 50 percent debt.[6] Without this access to funds the companies would not have been able to purchase additional hospitals as quickly or construct new hospitals as readily.

Convincing the investment and financial communities that high levels of debt are reasonable for the hospital industry has been a long, difficult struggle for the hospital management companies. The companies have argued that they can readily sustain such high leverage because of the predictability of their revenues. This predictability results from the steady demand for hospital services, the fact that the Medicare and Medicaid programs represent a virtual governmental guarantee of half their revenue, and the companies' ability to pass on increases of expenses through the cost-based reimbursement mechanism. It appears that the hospital management companies have convinced the analysts and investors; there has been a substantial increase in institutional ownership of the stock of these companies, and HCA, the largest company, has been the most highly leveraged "A"-rated industrial corporation in the country, as determined by both Moody's and Standard and Poor's credit rating services.[7]

The speed with which the investor-owned hospital firms have been able to mobilize funds has allowed them to capitalize on opportunities for growth and quickly arrange acquisitions. This ability has resulted from securing substantial bank lines of credit, borrowing funds in advance of need to have cash immediately available, and borrowing on the short term and later converting the debt to long term. The investor-owned companies' ready access to funds is not enjoyed by not-for-profit hospitals, which usually borrow for specific projects and experience delays before obtaining use of the funds.

The hospital management companies have benefited substantially from a favorable economic and regulatory environment. The investor-owned companies are heavily concentrated in the South and West, areas that have experienced significant population and economic growth in recent years. Of the beds owned by the five largest investor-owned firms, 73 percent are located in the South (especially Florida, Texas, Tennessee, and Kentucky) and 22 percent are located in the West (primarily California).[8] The growth of these areas has provided the companies with a steadily increasing patient base and has made them essentially recession-proof.

The South also is a region with little regulation of health care, providing a favorable environment for the hospital management companies to grow and prosper. The primary regulatory tool that affects the companies, certificate of need (CON) legislation, has worked to their advantage. CON has protected hospitals in many areas by making the entry of competitors difficult. By acquiring a hospital in a single hospital community, a company can secure a virtual monopoly in that market. Finally, the access to capital problems faced by the not-for-profit hospitals, coupled with rising costs, has provided the for-profit chains with an attractive source of candidates for acquisition.

The analysts also point to several other factors in the success of the management companies. The companies' hospitals are generally located in areas with a favorable payer mix, i.e., with relatively few Medicaid patients and a relatively high percentage of charge-based patients in relation to cost-based Medicare patients. Even with regard to the latter, for-profit companies have an advantage over the not-for-profit hospitals because the for-profit companies are reimbursed by Medicare for costs *plus* a return on equity. The companies also have been able to price aggressively and increase the intensity of care (and, thus, increase revenues) by purchasing sophisticated equipment and introducing new services. They have readily been able to pass on the increased costs of care (including interest expense) through the cost-based reimbursement mechanism and through higher charges, making them effectively immune to damage from inflation.

The benefits of economies of scale is another frequently cited reason for the success of the hospital management companies. The hospital sector has been one of the last remaining cottage industries, with each hospital operating independently. The hospital management companies have linked hospitals together to obtain economies of scale in financing, operations, and management systems. The combined earnings power and cash flow of the hospitals owned by the hospital management companies allow access to sources of financing that are not available to individual hospitals. Economies of scale in operations are also available to the hospital systems in the form of national purchasing contracts, shared equipment and services, and specialized design and construction assistance. The hospital chains can also attain economies of scale in systems development and usage through central services such as accounting, data processing, risk management, and internal consulting.

The final factor cited by analysts to explain the success of the hospital management companies is the quality of their management. As evidence of this quality, some analysts point to the foresight shown by the founders of these companies in entering the industry at an opportune time; in making attractive acquisitions; and in effectively overcoming difficult obstacles concerning credibility (profiting from sickness), financing (high leverage), and management depth. As further indicators of the continued quality and adaptability of management, they cite the companies' movement over time from an entrepreneurial orientation to a more professional management style without losing an innovative focus, their successful efforts to attract highly respected businessmen to their boards (with HCA as the prime example), and their ability to control their environment and plan for the future effectively.

Some analysts, however, are not convinced of the importance of management in explaining the past success of the hospital management companies. They feel that the highly favorable regulatory and economic situation that has existed in the industry could enable almost anyone to be successful. They refer to the fact that all the companies have performed extremely well as evidence of the failure-proof nature of the industry up until the present time. These analysts believe that although important differences in management ability exist among the companies the differences have not yet had a significant impact on relative performance.

Differences Among Companies

The analysts believe that the hospital management industry is more homogeneous than most other industries. However, they see among the companies some important differences that promise to become more crucial in the future. These differences relate to company image, financial policies, management style, operating philosophy, and strategic focus.

HCA, by far the largest company, is viewed as the most conservative and image conscious of the hospital management firms. It has made a concerted effort to win over the investment community by bringing in as chief executive officer Donald MacNaughton (the former chairman of Prudential Insurance), who is well respected by the investment and financial communities, and by attracting internationally known businessmen to its board of directors. HCA's board includes John deButts (former chairman of AT&T), Frank Carey (chairman of IBM), Owen Butler (chairman of Procter & Gamble), and Irving Shapiro (former chairman of DuPont).[9] HCA also has endeavored to assume the role of spokesman for the hospital management industry. In addition, HCA is distinguished by its decentralized operating philosophy and resulting emphasis on local hospital autonomy. The company is heavily involved in both owning and managing hospitals.

Humana is the most distinctively different of the companies. It is well known for its centralized operating philosophy, tight financial controls (i.e., strict measurement of revenue and expense performance), high leverage (although HCA is presently more leveraged due to its acquisition of Hospital Affiliates International) and aggressive management. Its clear focus is on the ownership of hospitals; it does not manage any hospitals under management contract. Humana also is hesitant to dilute its equity by issuing stock. Some view Humana as the most forward-looking and innovative of the companies and accordingly in the best position to respond quickly to economic changes and new opportunities.

NME's distinctive feature is its broad-based diversification. It is the only major hospital management company to own nursing homes and also has diversified into medical products and equipment distribution, construction services, purchasing services, and telephone answering devices.[10] NME (along with AMI) is heavily concentrated in California, compared with the southern region focus of the other companies. In addition, NME is the most financially conservative of the companies, having the lowest leverage.

AMI has more international interests than the other companies. It has developed a significant presence in the United Kingdom and other European nations. AMI is also known for the "unbundled" services that it sells to other hospitals. These services include laboratory, dietary and pharmaceutical services, respiratory therapy, mobile CAT scanners, and alcoholism recovery centers as well as the typical management services offered by most of the companies.[11]

Lifemark is appreciably smaller than the other hospital chains and has only recently been recognized as one of the major hospital management companies. Lifemark is especially strong in Texas, where it has grown rapidly. Lifemark also owns alcoholism recovery centers and dental labs.[12]

Acquisitions

Frequent acquisition of individual hospitals and, more recently, of other hospital chains has been a hallmark of the major hospital management companies. Securing attractive acquisitions has not always been easy for the companies. They have had to overcome the negative image of making a profit off the sick and of cream-skimming, the nervousness of the financial and investment communities about the high leverage of the companies, and the concern over the quality of care provided. The companies largely have been successful in countering these difficulties and have proven that they have the ability to make hospitals profitable. As a result, there is less reluctance among persons responsible for not-for-profit hospitals to having their hospitals purchased by one of the hospital systems. Individual hospitals even have begun approaching the hospital chains to solicit being acquired.

Competition among the companies for acquisitions has become quite heated. Prices paid per bed have risen to well over $100,000, sometimes approaching $250,000. The acquisition of other hospital chains has become more prevalent, having begun in 1978 when Humana doubled its size by means of the unfriendly takeover of American Medicorp (approximately $450 million for 39 hospitals with 7,838 beds).[13] Large acquisitions in the 1980s have included HCA's purchase of Hospital Affiliates ($650 million for 55 owned hospitals with 8,207 beds and 102 managed hospitals), General Care Corporation ($78 million for 8 hospitals with 1,294 beds), and General Health Services ($96 million for 6 hospitals with 1,115 beds), and AMI's acquisition of Hyatt Medical Enterprises ($69 million for 8 owned hospitals with 907 beds and management contracts with 26 hospitals) and Brookwood Health Services ($156 million for 9 owned hospitals with 1,271 beds and management contracts with 5 others).[14]

Success in the competition among the companies for acquisitions depends on two major factors: financial position (i.e., access to capital for making acquisitions) and reputation. A hospital management company must have the financial ability to make an acquisition. This involves considerations of how leveraged a company can become, how much stock it can issue, and how much cash flow would be available to support the acquisition once it is completed. For example, HCA was the only hospital management company that had the financial ability to pay the $650 million required to purchase a hospital chain the size of Hospital Affiliates.

Reputation as a factor in securing an acquisition can be of primary importance in some situations. All of the five major hospital chains seem to have good reputations regarding quality of care. Service expertise is another aspect of reputation where the chains do not differ significantly. Management philosophy and compatibility, however, are components about which there is considerable variation among the firms' reputations. Humana has been burdened with an unfavorable image as a result of its takeover of American Medicorp after which Humana dismissed a large number of American Medicorp executives and dismantled the company's management contract and nonhospital operations. Humana's loss to AMI in 1981 of Brookwood Health Services after an intense bidding war has been attributed to this image. Commenting on Humana's unsuccessful attempt to acquire Brookwood, *The New York Times,* stated that:

> Humana, Inc. has a reputation for dismissing the management of companies it takes over. Humana takes no prisoners has become a widespread comment among industry competitors and analysts. It is that reputation that apparently disturbed Brookwood Health Services, Inc. For several weeks Brookwood has actively fought what it considers a hostile takeover bid from Humana, and encouraged the entry of a white knight into the fray.[15]

Humana's centralized operating philosophy and tight financial controls have also contributed to the hesitancy of hospitals to be acquired by the company. This contrasts with HCA's decentralized operating style that allows individual hospitals to have more autonomy, thus making HCA a more attractive suitor to potential acquisition candidates. It is interesting that, although HCA phased out a large number of Hospital Affiliates's executives following the acquisition, it managed to do so in a manner that did not tarnish its reputation. NME and AMI have also developed favorable reputations as merger partners.

Making Hospitals Healthier

Once having completed acquisitions, the hospital management companies have demonstrated a remarkable ability to rejuvenate distressed hospitals and turn them into profitable operations. The analysts believe that several factors contribute to this success: economies of scale, financial sophistication, selection of services, marketing, and strategic planning.

The economies of scale come from being able to eliminate a portion of the fixed costs at an individual hospital when it becomes part of the system. The companies offer an individual hospital a variety of central management services, such as purchasing, accounting, data processing, risk management, and design and construction. The companies are also able to cut other aspects of the hospital's administrative overhead and can often reduce the overall staffing of the hospital by as much as 20 to 30 percent.

The companies provide an individual hospital with a financial sophistication that was not previously available to it. This includes ready access to capital for renovation and improvements, the ability to maximize reimbursement and collect lost charges through proved financial systems, and the ability to budget realistically and compare performance with the other hospitals in the system. In addition, the acquired hospital becomes subject to the financial control and operating discipline of the hospital system.

The hospital management companies also act to improve the profitability of the mix of services at the hospital. This may entail emphasizing the profitable services (e.g., surgical services as opposed to medical services, ancillary as opposed to routine services, simple as opposed to complicated operations, etc.), increasing the intensity of care with new services and technology, and adapting the services offered to be more consistent with the demographics of the hospital's market area.

Effective marketing requires efforts directed at physicians, patients, and the community with the objective of improving the hospital's image and broadening its patient base. The hospital chains place considerable emphasis on attracting new physicians and taking good care of those with existing privileges, recognizing that they are true customers of the hospital. Reduced rent for office space, access to high-technology equipment, and guaranteed incomes are just some of the techniques that have been used to attract physicians. The companies are particularly interested in attracting physicians who handle a preponderance of charge-based patients under the existing reimbursement system. The investor-owned companies also strive to improve the perception of the quality of care at the institution to increase patient and physician acceptance. The introduction of such amenities as color TVs, private baths, and special meals; an emphasis on cleanliness; and the attempt to reduce waiting time for emergency treatment, tests, operations, and the like are all efforts to improve conditions that are readily noticed by patients and physicians.

Finally, the hospital chains bring strategic planning to the hospital. This permits the hospital to analyze demographic trends, respond more effectively to changes, identify its competitive strengths and weaknesses, and find or develop its appropriate niche in the market.

Outlook for the Future

What is the outlook for the hospital management companies? The sell side analysts generally agree that the future looks bright. They expect a continued consolidation of the hospital industry, which will provide the hospital chains with the chance for increased market penetration. The analysts also foresee an opportunity for the companies to improve their profitability through operating leverage by raising the comparatively low levels of occupancy in their existing hospitals. The inherent advantages of hospital chains or systems in obtaining capital, realizing economies of scale, and utilizing effective marketing are anticipated to become more pronounced in coming years.

In addition, the quality of management is expected to assume greater importance as economic challenges increase. An industry shakeout may be in the offing, with the companies having the best management pulling clearly ahead of the others. The future also presents new opportunities for the hospital companies to become involved with alternative health care delivery systems (e.g., HMOs, primary care centers, freestanding emergency rooms, surgery centers). The companies could stand to benefit greatly by playing a leading role in the development of these alternative systems. However, they also have much to lose. The new forms of health care promise a negative effect on existing hospital business and provide more competition for the for-profit hospital companies.

There are several other factors that concern analysts in looking at the future of the hospital management companies. The future path of national and state health care regulation creates the most anxiety for the analysts. Whatever form regulation takes is expected to make it tougher for the hospital companies by forcing them to concentrate on cost control and possibly to subsidize the costs of other hospitals for teaching programs and for medical care for the poor. The analysts feel, however, that even with some form of strict prospective reimbursement the hospital management companies will be in the best position to cope of anyone in the hospital sector. High interest rates, the aging population causing an increase in less profitable cost-based patients, and antitrust considerations (as evinced by the U.S. Department of Justice's concern about the HCA acquisition of HAI) are other factors of concern to the analysts, who caution against assuming that the for-profit companies can do no wrong. Despite these concerns the analysts remain generally convinced of the attractiveness of the hospital management industry and its future growth potential.

References and Notes

1. The projects resulted in case studies on Humana and Hospital Corporation of America prepared by Richard Siegrist and issued by Harvard Business School Case Services

2. Company 1981 Annual Reports and 10Ks.

3. *The Wall Street Transcript*, March 9, 1981, pp. 26-27.

4. Hospital Corporation of America Prospectus, July 17, 1981.

5. Company 1981 Annual Reports.

6. Ibid.

7. *Answers to Questions Often Asked About HCA*, Hospital Corporation of America, 1982, p. 2.

8. Company 1981 10Ks.

9. Hospital Corporation of America 1981 Annual Report.

10. National Medical Enterprises 1981 Annual Report.

11. American Medical International 1981 Annual Report.

12. Lifemark 1981 Annual Report.

13. Humana 1981 Annual Report.

14. Company Annual Reports, 10Ks, and Prospectuses.

15. *The New York Times*, April 17, 1981, p. D3.

When Investor-Owned Corporations Buy Hospitals: Some Issues and Concerns

Jessica Townsend

When an investor-owned hospital chain buys a hospital it means many different things to many different people. To an administrator it may mean loss of a job. To a radiologist it may mean new equipment. To a county official it may mean the lifting of a financial burden from the county tax revenues, and to some patients it may mean a new and better-run hospital or fear of loss of access to services. But whatever the implications, for-profit corporate chains are buying hospitals from other chains, from proprietors that owned a single hospital, from counties, and from nonprofit corporations. Investor-owned corporations also contract to provide management services for nonprofit hospitals. These managed hospitals are often prime candidates for purchase at a later date.

The purchase of hospitals, particularly of nonprofit hospitals, by investor-owned hospital chains has raised questions that touch on ethics, law, research, medical education, costs, productivity, and more generally on how the public interest is being served. Over the past decade analysts have started to study some of the effects of such hospital purchases. But little information is now available about how such changes in ownership may be viewed by the various affected parties, whose attitude toward the change may in turn affect any number of factors, including both the purchase negotiations themselves and the policies under which the hospital will operate. This paper reports on an exploratory effort to learn more about the attitudes

51

and concerns of a range of interested people and the reactions of the purchasing corporations—how they responded to the concerns expressed and to what extent various interested parties were able to affect corporate actions.

Although time and resources did not permit a large-scale, systematic study, this exploration was undertaken to develop some preliminary information about the range of views of people who have been directly involved in recent sales of hospitals to investor-owned chains.

For this study, we identified the hospitals that were listed in the 1980 American Hospital Association *Guide* as being nonprofit or governmentally owned (city or county) and that were listed in the 1981 *Guide* as investor-owned. By cross-checking these 28 hospitals with the list in the directory of the Federation of American Hospitals (the trade association of the investor-owned hospitals) we were able to identify hospitals that had been purchased by one of the major investor-owned chains in 1981. One hospital bought by each of four companies was selected. Although our ability to obtain data on geographic diversity was limited by the fact that virtually all the hospitals identified were in sun-belt states, the selected hospitals were in four different states. The final selection of hospitals was influenced by the availability of key individuals during August 1982 when the interviews took place.

In each case the author attempted to contact, by telephone, the local health systems agency, a local newspaper, relevant public interest groups, the medical society or hospital association, one or two physicians (preferably the chief of staff or medical director), the administrator on the job before the purchase, a member of the hospital board, and county officials. In most cases we were successful in obtaining four to six interviews. (See the appendix to this paper for a list of the types of persons interviewed in each case.) In these informal interviews information was sought about the general background and reasons for the sale; the anxieties or concerns, if any, of the person being interviewed and whether (and how) these concerns had been addressed by the corporation or others; and what concerns they heard from others involved in the change.

We also examined one case in which a proposal for corporate takeover of a hospital did not go through. We included this case for the contrasts it provided with the cases in which the purchase was concluded.

It seems likely that the telephone interviews elicited only part of the picture. Although people were asked about their individual concerns, their responses were usually couched in somewhat global or public interest terms. A lot was heard about maintaining the quality of care, ensuring care for needy people, and attracting new physicians to underserved areas, but the respondents said nothing about how a change to corporate ownership affected them financially, why a politician was especially concerned about pleasing a specific constituency, or what the passing of control to a corporation really meant to the persons who yielded control. In short, we suspect that although we heard some genuine concerns, there may have been other concerns of a more personal nature that were not mentioned. The respondents were, after all, talking on the telephone to a stranger.

Clearly, a sample of five cases is so small as to preclude generalizing to all corporate purchases of hospitals. But even among the sample cases there were patterns of agreement on the topics that concerned people in similar positions. For example, hospital employees were always concerned about job tenure and benefits packages. However, in each case, the local situation produced its own set of concerns—e.g., about a deteriorating plant in need of replacement or, in the case of county hospitals, care for medically indigent people.

The Five Cases

County Hospital A

County Hospital A, a 270-bed general hospital in a small town 22 miles from the state capital and major medical centers, applied for a certificate of need (CON) in 1977 to replace its obsolete plant. Ever since, county officials had been involved in negotiations to raise the necessary capital for construction. Two attempts to issue general obligation bonds for a new hospital were rejected in a county-wide referendum. After the failure of the second referendum the local chamber of commerce studied the available alternatives and concluded that total replacement was required to bring the hospital up to date and that selling to an investor-owner was the best available option. The hospital board, hospital medical staff, and the county council all concurred with the decision.

A committee composed of members of the chamber of commerce and representatives of the hospital administrative and medical staffs was formed to review bids received from six investor-owned corporations. Three finalists were chosen, and the committee undertook a thorough investigation of the hospitals owned by these corporations. The committee, at the county council's expense, visited numerous sites where the corporations owned hospitals similar to County Hospital A; talked to local elected officials, community representatives, and medical staff; and reviewed hospital records. Committee members unanimously agreed that the corporation that offered the best financial proposal also scored best in meeting community and medical interests at the hospitals it already owned. Detailed negotiations were begun with that company.

During this period of decision and investigation, numerous concerns arose, including some opposition from senior citizens' groups and politicians. Opposition to the sale of the hospital was quieted by discussion with the groups and people involved, and the concerns of others (such as the hospital staff) were addressed during negotiations.

The major concerns and the way they were handled were as follows:

1. Care for the medically indigent—the proceeds from the sale of the hospital were placed in an escrow account, with the income to be used to reimburse the hospital at 90 percent of charges for people certified as medically indigent according to criteria developed by the county council.

2. Construction of a replacement hospital—the corporation agreed to build a replacement facility within three years.

3. Hospital employees—the corporate benefit package was generally satisfactory. The county agreed to fund accrued sick leave that would have been lost in the change-over. Continued employment was guaranteed by the corporation for a specified time.

4. Control of the hospital—although the corporation assumed ultimate control, an advisory board was set up with representatives from the community, hospital medical and administrative staffs, and the corporation.

5. Continuation of ambulance service—the corporation agreed to buy and operate the existing ambulance service.

6. Costs—it was recognized that costs of receiving care would increase, but the existence of other medical centers 20-30 miles away was thought to exercise a competitive restraint ensuring that cost increases would not be excessive.

7. Quality of care—the concern for maintaining quality of care was significantly lessened by the committee's investigation of other hospitals owned by the purchasing corporation.

It is notable that the medical staff of the hospital, with only one exception, voted for the sale. The area suffered from a shortage of physicians, and it was impossible to attract them to the old hospital. One year after the sale there were more than 10 new physicians practicing in the community. The chief of staff commented that the hospital plant was in great need of replacement and that the old administration was terrible and would not have made needed improvements: "I've been grinning ever since I heard of the sale. The patients are taken care of. The corporation makes its profit—that's what America is made of."

County Hospital B

County Hospital B is a 200-bed general hospital in a small town in a rural area about 1 hour's drive from a major metropolitan area that has a number of large medical centers. The town's population is served by a large multispecialty clinic that provides 130,000 patient visits a year from 36 physicians who staff the hospital and by two family practice clinics. The hospital receives referrals from a 9-county rural area, which includes some counties federally designated as medically underserved, and has an affiliation with a large medical school where local physicians teach and whose students and residents rotate through the hospital. County Hospital B, built in 1952 with Hill-Burton funds, was owned by the county.

When sale of the hospital was contemplated, it was rapidly becoming obsolete. An infusion of capital was needed to meet life safety codes, maintain accreditation, and purchase equipment needed to attract more physicians to the area.

The hospital board appointed 15 task forces to investigate the operations of the hospital and community health care needs. After a year of study the task forces reported on the deficiencies in the hospital and noted that approximately $75 per day was being added to the hospital bills of insured or self-paying patients because 65 percent of admissions either were not reimbursed or were reimbursed at less than full cost.

A broad-based community committee was formed to study alternatives, including issuing tax or revenue bonds to raise funds for renovation, affiliating with a nonprofit hospital system, and selling to an investor-owned hospital corporation. Each alternative was studied for its ability to meet a set of concerns that included obtaining adequate capital, ensuring charity care, maintaining local control, not adding to taxpayer costs, and providing high-quality care. The committee recommended to the county commissioners, the hospital staff, and the hospital board that only the option of sale to an investor-owned corporation would produce enough funds and affect enough change to remedy the deficiencies of the system.

A number of investor-owned corporations submitted bids—local people describe the situation as a "seller's market"—and addressed the set of concerns developed by the committee. The committee visited corporate headquarters and hospitals controlled by the companies. Before negotiations were concluded, local opposition began to coalesce around the issues of cost, control, and care of indigents. A citizens' group—Save Our Hospital—tried to have the issue put to a county-wide referendum, and some politicians supported the movement against corporate purchase. The local newspaper came out in favor of the purchase and set up an action-line phone number to respond to questions. As the proposed purchase became more controversial, medical and county leaders, businessmen, and city fathers united behind a public information campaign designed to reassure the people that local concerns were understood and to prevent misconceptions from developing. Although this campaign apparently reduced public concern, more important in concluding negotiations was the fact that a majority of the county commissioners were in favor of a sale.

The major concerns and the way they were addressed were as follows:

1. Indigent care—the corporation purchased the nonstructural assets of the hospital. Half of the proceeds of the sale were transferred to a nonprofit foundation set up by the county commissioners. The corpus of the capital was to be maintained in perpetuity with the earnings used to pay for charity care and the other community health needs. The foundation can also tap other nonprofit sources of financing.

2. Upgrading the hospital—the corporation agreed to upgrade the hospital to ensure accreditation and to start constructing a new hospital. Until construction is completed, the corporation will lease the old hospital. The old building will remain under county ownership and will be used for community services after completion of the new hospital.

3. Hospital employees' tenure and benefits—six months' tenure for all employees (except the administrator, who had antagonized some of the medical staff) was guaranteed. The corporate benefit package was acceptable to employees.

4. Control—the corporation was responsive to a desire to maintain local control as far as possible. The membership of the new advisory board is almost identical to the old board, and operating policies rest with them except for overall budget approval, which rests with the corporation.

5. Costs—the corporation agreed to maintain charges at a level commensurate with those of similar hospitals in the area.

Doctors Hospital

Doctors Hospital is a 165-bed general hospital in a metropolitan area of 1.2 million people. The city is served by 15 hospitals that have a total of more than 5,000 beds and is considered by the local Health Systems Agency to have an excess number of hospital beds. Only two hospitals have outpatient departments—Doctors Hospital is not one of them—with care for medically indigent people provided by a charity hospital system. The area is described as highly competitive for medical services.

Doctors Hospital, which is affiliated with two local nursing schools but no medical school, was a financially healthy, nonprofit institution owned by six doctors who thought that the future of small hospitals was uncertain, particularly in light of increasing costs and the demands of government regulation. The owners, who had been approached over the years by a number of investor-owned corporations, had no negative feelings about for-profit ownership because other hospitals in the area seemed to be providing quality care under investor ownership. However, the owners did not enter negotiations until 1980.

The sale seems to have been concluded with a minimum of fuss and concern, in large part because the purchasing company had a good reputation from its operation of other local hospitals. The hospital administrator and admitting physicians observed that the corporation "doesn't want to make all their hospitals conform to a corporate mold," that it maintains past board policies and allows the new community advisory boards a wide area of discretion, and that it preserves the quality of care and "does not wring out the last penny of profit."

The hospital administrator and medical director acted as the principal channels of communication between the corporation and hospital staff. Their knowledge of the corporate operations and verbal assurances from the buyer helped to quiet anxiety expressed by the hospital staff at a series of meetings.

The benefits expected from corporate ownership include improved management and financial reporting systems, access to corporate purchasing expertise and discounts, and new equipment.

Osteopathic Hospital

Osteopathic Hospital, with 81 beds, is located in a resort area 15 miles from another osteopathic hospital and in an area considered by the local health planning agency to have a surplus of hospital beds. It was a family operation that had been handed down from father to son. The physician-owner had obtained a CON to add beds despite opposition from the local health planning agency. (Some say the CON was obtained to make the hospital attractive to purchasers.)

The sale of Osteopathic Hospital took place so rapidly and quietly that the local newspaper and Health Systems Agency knew nothing about it until it was completed. The administrator said that negotiations took about two months, during which he talked to staff of the operations division of the purchasing company in a general way about maintaining the quality of care. A physician, who shortly after the sale became chief of staff, said: "No one knew it was being bought. The buyers didn't even inspect it during the daytime."

The speed and secrecy of the sale left little time for most people to be concerned about its impact before the fact. However, after the sale numerous concerns were expressed. The former chief of staff felt "betrayed" by an owner who said he would never sell the hospital. He contends that the staff have been reduced, some having been cross-trained to do two jobs. Good nurses have left because they saw their patient loads increasing, he said, and equipment that broke down was not repaired, roofs were leaking and not being repaired, prices were increased, and decisions were made at the corporate headquarters. This doctor said he will no longer admit patients to Osteopathic Hospital—a decision facilitated by a recent change in policy by other local hospitals, which now accept admissions from osteopathic doctors. It is reported that other medical staff also have decreased their admissions to Osteopathic Hospital and that the new administration is "bending over backwards to get doctors with private paying patients."

The previous owner tried to convince doctors that the purchase was in their best interest, and the corporate regional director has spent time with department heads and other staff to reassure them about continuity of tenure and quality of care, but with less than total success. The medical staff had waited for years for a renovation and expansion program. In spite of assurances by the company that construction will start, some are still skeptical and waiting to see bricks and mortar.

Suburban County Hospital

Suburban County Hospital is a county-owned and -operated facility that, according to county council staff members, is mired in layers of bureaucracy and suffering from bad administration. Recently the county executive sought to lease the hospital to an investor-owned hospital chain—a plan that failed, in large part because of community concerns and county council opposition. Some observers thought that political insensitivity by the politically ambitious county executive was a contributing factor, but it was also noted that some opponents of the plan were long-time political opponents of the county executive.

Prompted by the growing demands of the hospital on the county budget, the county executive sent a request for a proposal to several hospital management companies and received three responses—one from a nearby nonprofit hospital and two from investor-owned corporations. One of the corporations was selected, and a detailed leasing arrangement was developed. According to a county council staffer, the first the council knew about it was when the leasing plan was announced at a press conference. This was followed by an attempt by the executive to push the deal through under emergency legislation. The lack of council involvement in developing the lease and a feeling that the legislation was being ramrodded served to antagonize council members. They killed the legislation and proceeded to a detailed examination of the lease and of the corporations' operations. At the same time, public opposition to the lease was developing, and a coalition of consumer interest groups was formed.

The concerns expressed by the county council and the consumer groups were essentially the same. A major worry was whether the hospital would continue to provide care for medically indigent patients. Although the county earmarked money for indigent care and the lease contained assurances, doubts remained about whether the company would continue the full range of services currently provided and whether staffing would be maintained at acceptable levels.

A second major concern was that, although the agreement contained provisions for the hospital to be returned after a number of years to county control if desired, the money from the lease would not be sufficient to cover the cost of those parts of the hospital that would have been bought by the company. In addition, the county executive had described the lease as producing a financial bonanza for the county, when in fact the lease money had to be held for possible future repurchase of the hospital. There were other concerns—a monitoring commission was to be established but was described by the leader of the coalition of consumer groups as having "no teeth"; the loss of local control was disturbing to some; many details of the lease raised questions, such as including county health department premises in a building to be taken over by the corporation; and cost increases were feared to be excessive.

On the other hand, physicians on the hospital staff were generally pleased with the prospect of corporate management, mainly because it was thought that any change would be an improvement on the current situation. Physicians reported having had undue problems getting contracts through the bureaucracies; the hospital was included in county hiring freezes, consequently nursing shortages developed; the hospital used the county's computer system but had low priority, so billing was slow, resulting in frequent cash flow problems; obsolete equipment was not replaced; and purchasing went through the county system where specified items were sometimes changed. Physicians also were pleased that they would be represented on the proposed advisory board, whereas they had no policy role under the county ownership.

The leasing idea was finally abandoned, although an alternative scheme under which a nonprofit corporation would be established to run the hospital continued to be considered. Although many details of the arrangement are similar to the proposed lease to the for-profit company, the new scheme seems to have more community support, in part because local control is retained and in part because it is viewed as a community response to a community problem. The physicians and the county medical society support the new plan for the same reason they supported the former proposal: Any change has to be for the better.

Major Issues

Although many of the concerns expressed about a corporate takeover of hospitals were amorphous or ill defined (Will it be run as a business or a hospital? We really wonder what the corporate style will be.), concerns about several more specific topics arose in almost every case. These issues will be discussed below together with the ways the issues were resolved and the positions of the people who expressed concern about each issue.

Control

Every time a hospital chain buys a hospital there is a change in the locus of control—from a community board, county authority, or physician group to the corporation. Questions about the effects of the increasing penetration of the profit-making hospital chains into the control of health care facilities are being heard with increasing frequency.

The research for this paper sought to better understand who cared about the transfer of control when a hospital was purchased, what the nature of their concern was, and what was done to diffuse any anxieties that were expressed.

Although the hospitals studied were all nonprofit, they exhibited several different types of ownership and control before the purchase. One hospital owned by a nonprofit corporation was described to us as owned by the doctor and his family. Although this hospital had a 14-person board composed of physicians and community representatives, such as businessmen, bankers, and dentists, it was said that the hospital was very much a one-man business with the reins firmly held by the "owner." Another hospital was owned by a public facility authority but was leased to a group of physicians who, in effect, owned the hospital. Its governing board was composed of the five leasing physicians and the hospital administrator. In other cases, county authorities owned and operated hospitals, and boards of trustees were structured to include representatives from various sectors of the community and from health care providers.

In every case, after the purchase a new advisory board was created that typically included representation from physicians, the corporation, and the community. If the hospital was previously owned by the county, the county council retained the right to appoint the community representatives.

Numerous people said that the devolution of ultimate control of their hospital to the corporation had been a matter for concern. However, the nature of the expressed concerns varied, often with the position of the speaker. County council members or county commissioners expressed concerns about the loss of local control; physicians who had previously had representation on a board of trustees were concerned that their input into decisions might be diminished; community groups that became involved in the hospital purchase issue were interested in the effect on the overall mission of the hospital—an issue similar to the loss of local control but dealing more particularly with the range of services offered to specific elements in the population. In the case of Osteopathic Hospital, the doctors were worried about a change in mission; they were anxious to preserve the hospital for osteopathic medicine.

In one case, physicians expressed pleasure in the change. This was at a county hospital where the physicians believed that under the old administration they had not had enough voice on the board. With physicians representing one-third of the membership of the new advisory board, there is a feeling that their position has improved.

Enthusiasm about the change was the exception rather than the rule. More often, medical staff were concerned that decision making at the corporate level might diminish the impact of physicians on policies. However, after one year of for-profit ownership at the hospitals studied, most physicians appeared content with their relationship with the company, perhaps, because as one administrator commented, the company viewed the physician as much as the patient as the client. In only one of the four hospitals that were sold were the physicians upset by the change of control, saying that decisions are now made at corporate headquarters with the new administration functioning as "puppets." In that hospital physicians reportedly had not been able to organize to put pressure on the company, and the advisory board was said to lack influence.

Generally, the responsibilities of the new hospital advisory boards were said by those interviewed to be ill defined, but, because the new corporate owners were seen as trustworthy, most people felt that overall policy would emanate from the board and that the experience to date had been satisfactory. In two cases the board submits a budget to the corporation, and in each case the first budget had been approved. One respondent commented that: "We know that when a corporation invests they are going to call the shots—we gave it [control] up when we sold." But others commented that the advisory board directs the hospital much as the old board of trustees did.

However, despite the high level of expressed trust, in most cases the original owners had negotiated with the corporation to write into the sale contract some assurance of continuity of the hospital's mission. For example, one county hospital secured an agreement that the hospital would not become a specialty facility and that it would maintain such services such as obstetrics and emergency care.

In sum, although loss of local control was initially a concern and most people understood that loss of autonomy was inevitable, a year after the sale it was generally felt that the company could be trusted to be responsive to the advisory boards' recommendations and that there would be no insurmountable problems.

Job Security and Benefits

In all cases administrators expressed anxiety both about their personal job security and about the tenure of all hospital staff. Benefit packages were mentioned as being high on the list of staff concerns.

These cases suggest that job security for the top administrator is a well-founded concern. In three of the four hospitals that were sold, the corporations installed a new administrator. In one case, however, this was at the request of the old board of trustees, which asked that the company install one of their top administrators; everyone we talked to was delighted with the outcome. The former administrator, who had lost the support of the board and medical staff as well as that of community groups who viewed the hospital as being badly administered, was subsequently hired by the corporation.

A change in personnel at the top level of administration was apparently accepted by most people as part of doing business with corporations, because in all cases the seller negotiated with the buyer, as a condition of purchase, to get a certain amount of security for the remainder of the hospital staff. In each case there was an agreement that all staff would be retained for a certain period of time, ranging from a week to a year; thereafter, staff would be judged on competence. One hospital negotiated an assurance that any staff judged to be redundant would be offered training for another job in the hospital.

In all but one case everyone we spoke to expressed satisfaction that the sale had resulted in only a low level of staff turnover. "The corporation needs us, and we have good people" was one comment. The exception was Osteopathic Hospital, where the chief of staff expressed deep dissatisfaction with the way things had been handled. He contended that the number of staff fired was higher than he expected; that people who did not "fit the corporate pattern" were let go; that morale was low, despite efforts by the corporate regional director to assure the staff that all capable employees would be retained; and that the best nurses had left, partly because they were overworked and partly because they felt insecure about their jobs.

Benefit packages, although they had been a matter of concern before the sale, turned out to present no problems. Hospital administrators examined the company's benefits in detail and in general found them satisfactory—better than the existing package in some aspects, not as good in others.

Plant and Equipment

A need to replace the hospital plant was the prime reason for the sale of the two county hospitals, and a guarantee that this would be initiated promptly was made a condition of purchase in both cases. The county authorities had looked into other methods of achieving the same result and, despite an initial reluctance, decided that sale to a corporation was the most practical option. The ability of corporate enterprise to make capital expenditures was described as a crucial part of the decision to allow the hospitals to be absorbed into the investor-owned sector.

Many of the physicians interviewed expressed an interest in ensuring that obsolete equipment would be replaced and that state-of-the-art technology would be introduced. However, as far as we could determine, no specific promises were made to supply particular equipment at the request of physicians. However, in a more general way, physicians felt that the companies would do whatever was necessary. This confidence stemmed both from the notion that the particular company was a good one and that running a hospital in a competitive environment requires attention to the condition of equipment—it is part of good management practice. As one physician said: "The fear is that corporations always look to the bottom line, so my fear was that cost-effectiveness decisions would override other concerns, and some equipment is needed even if it isn't cost effective. But corporations know that they are in a competitive market and have to do quality care."

As it turned out, the physicians' confidence appears to have been well founded in these cases. Several physicians observed that during the first year of corporate operations new equipment had been bought. In one case the entire radiology department had been reequipped and an application for a CON for a CAT scanner has been submitted to the health systems agency.

The corporate purchase of one rural hospital was cited as instrumental in attracting more than 10 physicians to an area reportedly in need of medical manpower. The promises of a new hospital building within 2 years and the partial renovation of the existing plant were sufficient to attract several specialists, including a cardiologist and neurosurgeon. Today the hospital has new, well-equipped departments to serve these specialists.

In only one case, Osteopathic Hospital, did the purchaser reportedly fail to implement its verbal assurances about renovation and new equipment. Some of those interviewed thought that the corporation might be having financial problems.

In general, if the need for a large expansion or replacement project is a major reason for a sale, as is often the case, the seller may want to require an explicit contractual obligation to perform from the buyer. Physicians who might have been expected to seek formal assurances that equipment would be purchased seem not to have felt a need to do so because they trusted market forces to influence corporate management and because they trusted the company to maintain quality.

Charges for Care

Physicians, county officials, and consumer groups mentioned that the cost of hospital care was a concern, but often this concern was couched more in terms of the general rise in hospital costs than in an expectation that company ownership would result in excessive increases in charges. In only one of the four completed purchases did anyone interviewed mention that this was a matter discussed with the hospital buyer. Although it never was explicitly stated, there often seemed to be a feeling that the cost of care was not a topic on which the seller could negotiate and that this was one area of control that would inevitably be lost because, after all, the hospital was being sold to a profit-making business. Several themes that ran through the interviews were related to cost—e.g., that the company had been carefully looked at by the seller and was deemed to act responsibly and that hospitals function in a competitive environment and cannot price themselves out of the market if they want to survive.

After approximately one year of corporate ownership there seemed to be general acceptance of the increases in charges that had occurred. Even in a hospital where a 30 percent increase had reportedly taken place, people commented that there is no way of knowing if this was a greater increase than would have taken place under the old ownership. Because our investigations did not reveal how prepurchase charges compared with other local or national averages, the magnitude of change that would be needed to bring or keep each hospital in line with others cannot be determined.

A case in which cost negotiations came to light was the proposed leasing of Suburban County Hospital to a hospital management company. Suburban County Hospital is located in a state that has an active hospital rate review commission. The commission gave the company assurances that it would not lower the rates for 5 years even if the company significantly reduced costs; some county council members thought this was unfortunate because they wanted protection against increases not decreases. A representative of the local medical society suggested that the corporation would have no need to increase charges because the hospital had been so badly run by the county that operating costs could be substantially reduced by making some obvious and simple improvements in management. And it is from improved management that several of those interviewed about other cases hoped to see some impact on costs. The former administrator of one hospital, which in the year before it was bought had for the first time run a small deficit, said that savings from corporate purchases of supplies and equipment alone would be sufficient to put the hospital back in the black.

In sum, although charges for care are often a concern, they are frequently left to the company in the expectation that competitive forces, good management, and corporate integrity will restrain the rate of increase.

Quality of Care

Almost everyone, and particularly physicians and administrators, mentioned the importance of maintaining or improving the quality of patient care, and there seemed to be little fear that the corporate purchaser would undermine quality. Quality of care depends on so many factors, such as the quality of staff and equipment, the speed with which laboratory tests are completed, and the number of specialized services available, that it is difficult to discuss or negotiate about quality in general as an issue. However, many of the factors that contribute to quality care can be controlled or influenced by the corporation. The maintenance of plant, supplies, and equipment was not thought to present problems, and the general belief seemed to be that if those factors are well taken care of good physicians would be attracted to the hospital. Two other parts of the quality equation— nursing care and hospital staffing—were not included in the negotiations in these cases, except in the context of job security for existing employees. The expressed reason for the lack of anxiety about quality was, once again, that the sellers believed that their investigations of hospitals owned by the prospective buyer indicated that quality would be maintained. On the other hand, in the case in which such an investigation had not taken place—Osteopathic Hospital—a doctor commented that: "It's still a low-class hospital—the good staff have gone to other hospitals. I just saw costs going up and care going down, and I am not putting patients in there anymore." If others follow that course of action, as we were told is happening, Osteopathic Hospital may soon be in trouble. So, where there are competing hospitals, as many of our respondents indicated, there are incentives for the company to maintain or improve the quality of care.

Admission Policies

One of the most frequently made charges against the commercialization of the hospital industry is the practice of cream-skimming— seeking profitable patients and excluding patients who are poor and uninsured or who have complex illnesses. However, this issue was never brought up spontaneously by any of the people interviewed. When asked directly whether they had been concerned that the purchasing company might change admissions policies, the reply was always negative. This appears to be the result of a belief that the company would not interfere in the practice of medicine or that the physicians' influence would discourage the corporation from instituting policies of selective admissions.

County hospitals that had provided care to the medically indigent, and that had carried a significant amount of bad debt, went through complex negotations to ensure that poor people would continue to receive care. Three county hospitals were examined, two where the sale was completed and one where it was denied by the county council. In each case indigent care was the major issue for both the public and the county authorities; the failure of negotiations in one case occurred in part because many people felt that despite detailed arrangements written into the contract the provisions for enforcement were inadequate. In the cases of the two county hospital sales that took place, only the issue of replacing the hospital itself took precedence over the issue of indigent care. No doubt the concern was fueled by the active concerns of citizens' groups, but everyone from the hospital administrator to the county officials, from the newspaper editors to the physicians, said that indigent care was at the top, or close to the top, of their list of concerns.

Arrangements for financing care for medically indigent people involved setting up a fund with a portion of the proceeds from the sale and using the interest to pay for hospital care. Thus, the county would continue to pay for the care of the indigent. Negotiations with the corporation involved obtaining a guarantee that medically indigent people would not be denied admission to the hospital. In one case the county developed criteria to define indigency, and in another the purchaser agreed that the county would have to pay only 90 percent of customary charges for the care of the indigent.

Providing care for the population traditionally served by the county hospital was a requirement set forth by the county authorities, in most cases before detailed negotiations began, and did not become a matter for dispute in the cases in which a sale took place.

Buy-Back Provision

One further issue peculiar to the county hospitals was that the sales contracts included buy-back provisions if, after a specified period of time, the county was dissatisfied with the company's operation of the hospital. The details of the financial arrangements differed among the county hospitals examined, but for the two sales that went through they seemed satisfactory to the county authorities and interested citizens. In the case of the county hospital for which the corporate leasing arrangement could not be completed, both county council members and the leader of a citizens' coalition cited the buy-back arrangement as an unsatisfactory feature of the lease, which contributed to the failure of the proposal.

Although it may not be essential for a corporation to agree to buy-back arrangements, it appears important in reducing a seller's nervousness about the sale. Several people interviewed mentioned the topic spontaneously in the interviews.

The Process

Time and again interviewees said that, although other companies might act differently, they felt sure that the corporation purchasing *their* hospital would act with integrity. We heard this with reference to admission policies, staff policies, local autonomy, plant and equipment, and in general about behaving like a responsible health care provider rather than a profit-maximizing entity. We heard it from board members, county council members, administrators, and physicians. In some cases this belief was based on the fact that, before detailed negotiations with a company began, the sellers had looked closely at the corporate operations and at hospitals it owned. In other cases criteria were established that a purchaser would have to meet before being seriously considered. The result was that, in the hospitals that were sold, those involved felt that they were dealing with a known entity and they liked what they knew; adversarial relationships did not develop. Furthermore, it is possible that, because of this initial trust, topics that could have become issues did not and, thus, were not mentioned to us as being concerns. For example, when physicians and administrators did not mention physician contracts (such as are often arranged with radiologists and pathologists) as an area of concern, the interviewer asked about it. Most often the response was that the corporation was aware of existing contracts and obligations and that there had been no fears that a suitable arrangement would not be made. One wonders whether such a relaxed attitude would have been possible in the absence of trust.

In the one case where the sale was concluded without consultation with hospital staff and physicians and without an investigation of the company by representatives of the interested groups, the result was strikingly different. Various people commented that corporate management showed little concern for their problems, that staff morale was low, and that a general feeling of insecurity was current. In this hospital concern was expressed about admission policies and about the nature of a for-profit enterprise.

Other elements in the process of changing to ownership by a for-profit chain also may have been important. In some cases an impressive and time-consuming process was undertaken whereby committees were assembled to identify and analyze the alternatives to corporate takeover and to identify the major areas of public and internal hospital concern. The result was that a clear and public decision had been made that corporate ownership was the best available option and that the company selected would be responsive to public concerns. Here again the contrast with two places that omitted these steps—Osteopathic Hospital and Suburban County Hospital—is striking. In the case of Suburban County Hospital, it is particularly tempting to conclude that if the decision-making process had been more public—if the county council had been involved along with the county executive in selecting the corporation—the outcome might have been different. Only after the council was presented with the leasing proposal did its staff initiate the type of investigation of the corporation that in other cases preceded the negotiations. They looked at other county hospitals owned by the company and did not like what they saw; one council staff person stated that the findings of the investigation were "the killers." With greater political sensitivity and greater public involvement—in other words, greater attention to process—a corporate leasing arrangement under similar terms possibly would have been acceptable.

Conclusions

The outstanding impression gained from these cases and from conversations with people who had varied interests in them was that the takeover of these hospitals by for-profit chains often generated only low levels of anxiety. There were, of course, exceptions, but these appeared to be as much or more a matter of clumsy political maneuvering and lack of openness with the people involved than a matter of substantive concern that the company could not answer.

There were a few differences among the hospitals on which issues were important. For county hospitals the issues of indigent care, buy-back provisions, and cost generated considerable activity both by local politicians and by consumers who formed groups to make their positions public. In contrast to the sales of physician-owned (or controlled) nonprofit hospitals, a great deal of public discussion surrounded the sale of county facilities, with local newspapers, politicians, and community leaders becoming involved in disputes and with the purchase becoming a political issue. Participation in discussions of the takeover of the physician-owned facilities appears to have been confined to those directly involved with the hospital—owners, board, administration, staff, and physicians.

There were also clear differences in the interests of the various people with whom we talked, the interests being related to their position or relationship with the hospital. Although there were some exceptions, the expressed concerns of the different groups were as follows:

• Consumers—for the county hospitals, consumers became interested in the issues of indigent care, local input into hospital policies, and the financial deal, particularly buy-back provisions. There was no organized expression of consumer interests when physician-owned hospitals were bought. It was, however, noted that patients were aware of the changed status of their hospitals, often because the purchasing company mounted publicity campaigns. Physicians commented that the concerns expressed by their patients were over the prospect of increased charges. In general, the change was readily accepted.

• Board Members—Because the agreement of the hospital board had been obtained before detailed negotiations for the sale proceeded, there generally were few issues that concerned them by the time the sale took place. The topics mentioned as being of interest included quality of care and the status of the new advisory board.

• Administrators—Although administrators generally were involved in every aspect of negotiations from an early stage, two topics emerged as the focus of their concerns: staff job security and benefit packages. Maintaining the quality of patient care also was mentioned as a more general concern.

• Physicians—This group frequently expressed an interest in the quality of plant and equipment, an interest most often spoken of in terms of how the corporation could improve these conditions. Physicians were also concerned about quality of care in general and about ensuring that physicians' voices would be heard at the corporate level.

• Politicians—This group became involved only when a county hospital was being sold. Their areas of concern were similar to those of consumer groups: indigent care, local control, and cost. They were also concerned with the financial details of the sale, particularly how to finance indigent care from the proceeds of the sale and how to conserve capital for eventual possible buy-back.

Almost all people interviewed in connection with three of the five cases were well pleased with their new situation. Two cases were markedly different with considerable antagonism expressed. The difference between the two groups did not seem to be because of characteristics of the purchasing corporation or of the hospital being bought or of the people interviewed. To the extent we could understand it, the difference appeared to be in the process by which the idea was developed or by which the sale took place.

As mentioned in greater detail earlier, when the purchasing company had been investigated before the sale and the major concerns of interested groups had been brought out in the open, most doubts were dealt with before the takeover. Most people expressed an understanding and acceptance of the idea that the company had to make money off hospital operations. Few doubted that, because of certain external constraints, the company would have an interest in maintaining the quality of care and loyalty of staff. That is, if a hospital is to be profitable, it must attract good physicians and their patients and it must control costs. More positively, there were expectations that corporate management would benefit the hospital both through economies of scale and the introduction of specialized management techniques.

A number of people noted that during the year after the sale they were delighted with the new administration and with the resources that the corporation made available. These included sending management specialists to the hospital to deal with specific problem areas, the advice given by the corporate central office in such areas as purchasing, and the economies achieved through centralized buying. In short, if the groundwork was well done, the companies in these cases were not only accepted but were also warmly welcomed.

However, it must be kept in mind that each of these hospitals had experienced corporate ownership for only a year or so. The longer-run relationships between the corporate management and the medical staff; the community; board members; and administrative, nursing, and other staff could be not be explored. Equally, if not more important, the impact of corporate ownership on such matters as cost, quality of care, and the long-term existence of the hospitals was not investigated. These and other outcomes are of critical importance to the health care system of each locality in which an investor-owned hospital is active and to the nation's health care system as investor-owned hospital chains continue their expansion into health care delivery systems.

APPENDIX

PRINCIPAL INTERVIEWS CONDUCTED FOR THIS PAPER

1. County Hospital A
   Editor of local newspaper
   Former health systems agency staff person
   Admitting physician
   Physician member of hospital board
   County manager
   Former administrator of hospital

2. County Hospital B
   State Health Planning and Development Agency staff
     members
   Physician—member of task force and committee involved
     with negotiations of sale
   Lawyer for foundation created to fund indigent care
   Physician—member of advisory board
   Reporter on local newspaper
   Banker

3. Doctors Hospital
   Executive director—State Health Planning and Devel-
     opment Agency
   Executive director of area hospital council
   Administrator of hospital
   Medical director of hospital

4. Osteopathic Hospital
   Staff member of health systems agency
   Editor of local newspaper
   Former administrator of hospital
   Present assistant administrator of hospital
   Former chief of staff of hospital

5. Suburban County Hospital
   Executive director of local medical society
   Staff member of health systems agency
   Member of the county council
   Staff of councilman
   Director of local citizens' coalition
   Director of state rate review commission
   Admitting physician at hospital

Physician Involvement in Hospital Decision Making

Stephen M. Shortell

People in the future will need to learn organization the way their forefathers learned farming.

—*Peter Drucker*

Medical decision making is an organizational process. Even at the level of individual clinical judgment, a myriad of prior "organizational" decisions have been made that affect what appears to be an autonomous clinical judgment made by a trained professional. For example, a surgeon's choice of a given technique for a particular operation has been conditioned by prior decisions, such as the number and types of operating rooms available, types of equipment purchased, the quality and mix of surgical assistants and nursing staff, and the organization of the operating room schedule itself. The surgeon's decision may also be influenced by prior decisions made by the hospital's quality assurance committee. In brief, "micro" decisions involving individual clinical judgment and "macro" decisions involving larger organization-wide resource allocation and policy issues are highly interrelated. The nature of physician involvement in hospital decision making must be understood within this context.

There are five major themes to this paper. The first is that the major hospital decision makers—trustees; administrators; voluntary staff physicians; hospital-compensated physicians; and, increasingly, nurses—will view the decision-making process primarily as a function of their actual degree of involvement in the organization, the degree of involvement that they feel they should have, and the nature of the issue at stake. Physicians and nurses typically will be most concerned about decisions affecting patient care—the ultimate goal. Administrators and trustees, although also concerned about patient care, will focus most of their energies on resource acquisition and management issues—the instrumental goals for facilitating cost-effective patient care.

The second theme of this paper is that the distinction between "clinical" and "administrative" decision making is becoming blurred. New technology, regulation, and competitive forces are giving rise to a number of decisions in which no single professional group has controlling interest and participation by all groups is required.

The third theme is that physician involvement in hospital decision making is affected by whether the hospital is voluntary or investor-owned, a freestanding hospital or a member of a multi-unit system.* For example, a hospital that becomes part of an investor-owned chain may find its physicians more actively involved in hospital governing board activities than previously.

The fourth theme is that decision making may be moving away from the "dual authority" model of split administrative and clinical decisions to a more "shared authority" model based on increasing collaboration between administrators and physicians. This is partly because of the blurring of decisions noted above but is also due to a number of other factors that will be discussed.

The fifth theme is organized around some evidence that suggests that greater physician involvement in hospital-wide decision making is associated with lower costs and higher-quality care. In this context the relationship between cost containment and quality of care also is examined.

Where relevant, these themes are specifically considered for their implications regarding for-profit ownership of hospitals. This is particularly true in regard to the types of decisions faced, dual authority and shared authority decision-making models, and specific forms of physician involvement in decision making. At the same time it is important to recognize that the differences in economic orientation between for-profit and nonprofit hospitals may be narrowing, with some interesting implications for hospital behavior.

For brevity's sake, this paper will not describe the historical evolution of physician involvement in hospital decision making. The main concern here is with current developments and implications for the immediate future. The paper will not serve as an exhaustive review

---

* It is recognized that there are also important differences between teaching and non-teaching hospitals, but the primary focus of this paper is on ownership and system versus nonsystem differences.

of the literature. Rather, it will highlight some of the more significant studies and major findings.

This paper is divided into five major sections. First, the major kinds of decisions made by hospitals are described. Second, those individuals primarily involved in hospital decisions are noted, and two models of decision making are examined. Third, the nature of the involvement is highlighted. Fourth, evidence bearing on the relationship between physician/hospital decision making and the cost and quality of care is summarized. Finally, a number of future issues influencing physician/hospital decision making are discussed.

A Typology of Hospital Decision Making

A simple typology of decision making is shown in Table 1, which suggests that decision-making strategies used by hospitals depend on (1) the degree of agreement or certainty among the key parties as to their preferences for specific outcomes and (2) the degree of confidence or certainty in the cause-effect relationships involved—i.e., whether the decision will actually produce the desired results. For example, in the first cell where all parties agree on preferences about outcomes and the certainty of cause-effect relationships is relatively straightforward, decisions can be made on a fairly routine "computational" basis. Decisions involving the amount of standard supplies to keep in inventory in the hospital's central supply department serves as an example of a computational decision strategy. For the most part, physicians do not get involved in such decisions, which are primarily made by hospital support department heads and increasingly are being computerized or otherwise automated.

TABLE 1 A Typology of Physician/Hospital Decisions

| | | Certainty of Preferences about Outcomes | |
		Certain	Uncertain
Certainty of Cause-Effect Relationships	Certain	1 Computational	2 Compromise
	Uncertain	3 Judgmental	4 Inspirational

SOURCE: Adapted from Thompson, J. D. *Organizations in Action.* New York: McGraw-Hill, 1967.

The second cell involves situations in which there is certainty about cause-effect relationships but in which the parties involved disagree about desired outcomes. These decisions are labeled "compromise" decisions. For example, a hospital may be faced with the decision of whether to purchase a CT scanner or expand the laboratory department's capabilities. In either case the cause-effect relationships are known (the decision will most likely result in improved patient care), but the parties disagree as to the areas of hospital operation (radiology or lab) in which they wish to see the improvement. It is important to note that general economic forces, external regulation, and competitive pressures are increasing the number of compromise decisions that hospitals must make. These are situations where the efficacies of decisions are known but where there are insufficient funds to implement all of them. Compromise decisions are a major area of physician involvement in hospital decision making, as each specialty group strives to maintain or expand its scope of responsibility. Thus, for the most part, physicians become involved in these decisions in order to protect their interests.

The third cell involves situations in which preferences about outcomes are known and agreed upon but where there is uncertainty about the cause-effect relationships. These situations constitute "judgmental" decisions. For example, the decision to improve a hospital's financial position may be agreed upon by all parties, but uncertainty may exist about the best strategy or combination of strategies to accomplish this. Physicians are becoming increasingly involved in judgmental decisions but for a different reason than their involvement in compromise decisions. In compromise decisions they become involved primarily to protect their interests, but in judgmental decisions they become involved because their expertise as physicians is needed. For example, many administrators have relied heavily on physician advice in justifying major capital purchases or expansion projects to health systems agencies.

The fourth cell describes situations in which uncertainty exists about both preferences for outcomes and cause-effect relationships. These decisions are labeled "inspirational." For example, a rural hospital with low occupancy may be pondering whether to develop an ambulatory care program or affiliate with an urban medical center. In terms of cause and effect it is not clear that either option will increase admissions. Furthermore, with either option the parties involved may disagree about likely outcomes. To reduce the uncertainty surrounding such decisions, hospitals are increasingly adopting methods of formal environmental assessment and long-run strategic planning.

Their purpose is to transfer these decisions from the inspirational category to the judgmental or compromise categories. In this process medical opinion is becoming increasingly important, resulting in further physician involvement in hospital decision making.

Because new technology, regulation, and competition have given rise to a great number of compromise, judgmental, and inspirational decisions, physicians and administrators have found themselves more dependent on each other, and the distinction between clinical and administrative decision making is blurring. Three prototypical decision examples help illustrate the point.

The first example has to do with whether a hospital should expand its ambulatory care activities, perhaps by developing a satellite clinic or a health promotion program or by sponsoring a group practice. Although a number of marketing, planning, and related administrative considerations are involved in such a decision, clinical issues are intertwined throughout. These include issues of what kinds of patients will be treated, triage, specialty mix of the physicians involved, determination of clinical privileges, and the type of referral relationships to be established. A hospital's decision to expand its ambulatory care activities can often be controversial and divisive because it may directly threaten existing staff who are trying to maintain or expand their practices. Thus, the administrative and clinical considerations involved take on added importance.

The second example is represented by the question of whether to pay hospital-based specialists, such as pathologists and radiologists, a percentage of the gross revenues generated or a percentage of the net revenues generated. From an administrative and cost containment perspective, payment based on the percentage of gross revenue offers no incentive for efficiency, but payment based on the percentage of net revenue creates an incentive to contain expenses. However, economic and administrative considerations also must take into account some underlying clinical issues. These include the effect of the compensation method on the general quality of the staff in the laboratory and radiology departments, on the institution's ability to keep up with technological advances and to offer new tests and services desired by medical staff members, and on the general maintenance of the quality of care.

A third example is represented by the question of whether to change from team nursing, in which a group of nurses care for a group of patients, to primary care nursing, in which one nurse and often an assistant are assigned responsibility for managing a patient's care throughout the patient's stay. A variety of administrative and clinical issues are raised by such a decision. They include cost considerations, likely impact on turnover, absenteeism, job satisfaction, ability to recruit nurses, relationship with other departments, continuity of care, and quality of care. These issues are interrelated and difficult to separate, even though each group will approach the question from its particular area of concern—nurses from the perspective of job satisfaction and quality of patient care, physicians from their perspective of quality of care and how the change will affect nurse/physician relationships, and administrators from the perspective of costs and adequacy of staffing in addition to concerns about quality of care.

Other examples could be used to illustrate the blurring of administrative and clinical decision making. Some additional examples are provided in Table 2, categorized according to the computational, compromise, judgmental, and inspirational frameworks.

Although it provides some insight, the typology described above is oversimplified. At least two other sources of complexity appear to be important in understanding the nature of the hospital decision-mak-

TABLE 2   Examples of Physician/Hospital Decisions

1. Computational
     Maintaining inventory levels.
     Hiring ancillary staff.
     Hiring additional nurses to increase coverage.

2. Compromise
     Suspending privileges of a popular physician.
     Admitting a new physician in a specialty that is already well supplied.
     Purchasing a CT scanner or a major piece of lab equipment.
     Developing a new compensation arrangement for the director of the laboratory.

3. Judgmental
     Expanding physician continuing education efforts to improve quality of care.
     Hiring a full-time director of medical education to improve quality of care.
     Changing to computerized billing system.
     Establishing a long-range planning department.

4. Inspirational
     Adding a new clinical service.
     Developing a hospital-sponsored group practice.
     Affiliating with a medical school.
     Merging with another hospital.

NOTE: The examples are not necessarily mutually exclusive. They will obviously vary depending on people's perceptions of the cause-effect relationships and preferences for outcomes. They also depend on the stage of the decision-making process. For example, as more information becomes available, some inspirational examples may become compromise or judgmental decisions.

ing process. The first is the influence of differences in ownership of hospitals—particularly in regard to voluntary versus investor-owned hospitals and freestanding hospitals versus those belonging to multiunit systems. The second is the distinction between those matters in which physician and hospital interests coincide and those in which they are more likely to be in conflict.

A basic distinction between investor-owned and voluntary hospitals is the former's need to make a return on stockholders' equity. This return might be viewed as the ultimate goal of the investor-owned hospital with the rendering of patient care serving as an instrumental goal or means of achieving the ultimate goal of return on equity. In contrast, for the voluntary hospital the ultimate goal is the delivery of patient care to the community and generating a surplus (or profit) serves as an instrumental goal or means by which this is achieved. In brief, the means-ends relationships become reversed.

It is important to note that for both investor-owned and voluntary hospitals financial viability and the delivery of cost-effective patient care are important, whether as instrumental or ultimate goals. Nevertheless, one might hypothesize that this difference will affect the decision-making process and the resulting choices of specific services offered by hospitals. The investor-owned hospital will presumably be particularly interested in adding services that will increase return on investment. From the overall portfolio or mix of services provided by a hospital, the requirement for profitability provides a constraint on expansionary impulses. Voluntary hospitals under traditional cost-based reimbursement have been able to develop a wide range of services to meet community needs or demands. In recent years, with the growth of regulation and competition, voluntary hospitals have also had to become more selective in adding new services and programs. Thus, a more fine-grained analysis of decision-making differences by investor-owned and voluntary hospitals is required. The decision framework presented in Table 1 provides a context for such analysis.

Specifically, investor-owned hospitals are likely to face somewhat more computational and judgmental decisions, while voluntary hospitals are likely to experience somewhat more compromise and inspirational decisions. As will be recalled, in computational and judgmental decisions preferences about outcomes are more certain. This is more likely to be true in investor-owned hospitals both because they are a part of systems typically characterized by the centralized influence of corporate offices and because of the more homogeneous group of defined constituents in terms of stockholders. In contrast, voluntary community hospitals have many different constituents to serve. They also tend to have high turnover in upper administrative ranks, and, therefore, many lack strong continuous managerial direction. In brief, there are likely to be more debates about the preferences for different kinds of outcomes in voluntary community hospitals than in investor-owned hospitals. As such, in voluntary hospitals the decision-making process may be somewhat more complex and indeterminate than in investor-owned hospitals.

In general, hospitals belonging to a multi-unit system seem likely to be more involved in computational and judgmental decisions than are freestanding individual hospitals. This is due in part to the influence of a corporate headquarters office with greater managerial staff expertise, which can reduce the uncertainty of cause-effect relationships surrounding given decisions. Also, the presence of an overall corporate mission and value system can help orient individual hospitals toward achievement of more common objectives, resulting in less disagreement regarding desired outcomes. In contrast, individual hospitals, often lacking such expertise and direction, may become involved in more compromise and inspirational decisions. These suggested differences, however, also depend on other factors, including the maturity of the multi-unit system and its emphasis on innovation. For example, a multi-unit system in the early years of existence may face a greater number of compromise decisions as it attempts to gain agreement among member hospitals regarding overall directions. Furthermore, a system at the cutting edge is experimenting with new programs, services, and organizational arrangements and may thus face a high number of inspirational decisions. Decision-making strategies will also be influenced by the degree of centralization that exists between the corporate headquarters office and individual member hospitals. The suggested differences by ownership and system status are summarized in Table 3.

TABLE 3   Most Prevalent Types of Decision-Making Strategies, by Type of Hospital

Decision-Making Strategy	Voluntary Hospital	Investor-Owned Hospital	Single Hospital	Multi-Unit System Hospital
Computational		+		+
Compromise	+		+	
Judgmental		+		+
Inspirational	+		+	

Convergence versus Divergence of Interests

Determining where physician and hospital interests overlap and where they diverge is difficult because the relationship is subject to complex and rapidly changing forces. In general, hospital and physician interests coincide most often in areas involving expansion of hospital programs and services that are complementary rather than substitutable with physician services. Examples include increasing the number of beds; acquiring sophisticated technology, such as nuclear magnetic resonance scanners; and adding selected support services, such as occupational therapy, physical therapy, and social work, which are uneconomical for most physicians to incorporate into their private practices. Interests also coincide when physicians and hospitals can assist each other in responding to external regulation or changes in payment. A noteworthy example is the development of quality assurance committees in response to the establishment of Professional Standards Review Organizations (PSROs).

Conversely, hospital/physician interests diverge when physicians perceive the hospital to be in direct competition or when the hospital believes physicians are acting counter to the long-run objective of the hospital. Thus, as previously noted, hospitals' efforts to expand their ambulatory care activities may meet medical staff opposition because of fear of direct competition for patients and hospital beds.[2] Opposition may also be based on philosophical objections to the "corporate practice of medicine." Regulations or changes in payment also can create conflict rather than representing the "common enemy" against which hospitals and physicians can unite. For example, limiting hospital revenues by reimbursing on a case-mix basis may create conflict between a hospital's economic interests and the physicians' economic and professional interests.

It is important to note that there is frequently more disagreement among physicians than between physicians and hospitals. Physicians are not a unitary group and seldom act in concert on a given issue. Differences exist by specialty, years in practice, and geographical location, in addition to individual differences in personality and philosophy. For example, surgeons and other specialists are typically strong supporters of hospital ambulatory care programs because they usually benefit directly from increased referrals. Primary care physicians, in contrast, are likely to be the most vocal critics because of perceived competition. Even here, differences exist depending on the patients to be served. For example, if the primary purpose of an expanded ambulatory care program is to serve more Medicaid patients, private practice physicians may be supportive because of their desire to limit the number of Medicaid patients in their practice.

The diversity among physicians is important to recognize in considering decisions involving almost any new program, service, technology, or reorganization. In brief, each physician and specialty group will be concerned if the decision is likely to benefit other groups or interests more than their own. As Harris[3] notes, in the extreme, this results in

. . . each clinical service of the medical staff . . . striving to maintain and expand the magnitude of its own defensive position. . . . Each service gets its own intensive care unit. Each intensive care unit gets its own laboratory. The idea behind all of these arrangements is to insure the exclusive availability of a set of inputs to a small group of demanders. In that way no one is going to get bumped.

Although this often creates problems for hospital administrators and trustees, it also is to their advantage in that it facilitates "divide and conquer" strategies and affords administrators some flexibility in playing off the interests of one group of physicians against another. How these relationships are influenced by competition, regulation, and related factors is described in a subsequent section.

The Decision Makers

The most important point to understand about decision making in hospitals is that there is no single decision maker. Rather, decision making is a complex and often diffuse process involving multiple coalitions of key people, including physicians; administrators; trustees; and, increasingly, nurses. These coalitions exert different degrees of influence depending primarily on the topic. Typically, physicians exert the most influence over clinical matters, such as determining staff privileges, establishing practice protocols, reviewing quality of care, and determining patient admission and discharge. Executive-level administrators exert the most influence over hospital policy and planning activities particularly as they relate to the organization's external environment. Middle-level executives and department heads typically exert the most influence over matters related to daily staffing, budgeting, and procurement of supplies. The influence of trustees is primarily felt in the areas of long-run strategic planning and articulating the overall mission and direction of the hospital. Nurses are striving to become more involved in all of these areas. From this general description, it is possible to highlight two general "models" of decision making in hospitals: the dual authority model and the shared authority model.

The Dual Authority Model

The dual authority model is best developed by Pauly and Redisch[4] and Harris[5] and was first described by Smith.[6] In the Pauly/Redisch version the hospital is seen as a physicians' cooperative in which physicians' decisions largely determine the nature of hospital operations. The administration largely exists to provide the equipment, supplies, and facilities for physician use. Although two distinct lines of authority (administrative and clinical) are recognized, administrators seldom oppose physicians because the hospital's success and the administrator's own job security are closely tied to satisfying the demands of the physician staff.

In the Harris version the administrative and medical split is conceptualized as two different "firms." The medical staff constitutes a "demand division" and the administration a "supply division." Each division has its own managers, decision-making strategies, operating rules, and policies. Third-party payers recognize this separation in the form of separate payment policies for ambulatory care versus inpatient care. In brief, although hospitals and physicians are in fact involved in a joint production process, they are largely organized as separate entities; therein lies much of the difficulty in hospital decision making as it pertains to the allocation of scarce resources. Until recently, the "expert" power of the physician as legitimated by the state has dominated the decision-making process over the "legitimate" power (i.e., formal position authority) of the administration. Furthermore, physicians control both their own and the hospital's inputs. As Harris notes:

Doctors are in a position to deem all sorts of demands as necessary for their patients. This is not the same thing as saying doctors order useless tests to satisfy some ulterior motives. Additional demands for inputs above the hypothetical scientific minimum are going to be regarded by doctors as improvements in quality.[7]

The issues suggested by the dual authority model of decision making are more complex for voluntary hospitals than for investor-owned hospitals. If one assumes that the goals of investor-owned hospitals are somewhat more homogeneous and targeted than are the goals of voluntary hospitals, the interests of physicians and the hospital may be more closely aligned. In contrast, voluntary hospitals may pursue a variety of community objectives, not·all of which may contribute to financial viability and which may in fact detract from or even compete with physician interests. But as cost containment pressures continue, voluntary and investor-owned hospitals are becoming more alike in their orientation to financial viability. In single hospital communities, this may lead to further hospital competition with the medical staff. In multiple hospital communities where physicians have alternatives for admitting patients, hospitals are more likely to pursue initiatives that will complement rather than compete with staff interests.

The Shared Authority Model

The shared authority model is the product of recent developments. Briefly stated, it involves more conjoint[8] or shared decision-making power between administrators and physicians and increased integration of clinical and administrative information. This model has emerged as a result of legal, economic, and societal forces. From a legal perspective, the *Darling* decision[9] in 1965 established the hospital's ultimate legal responsibility for the quality of care. This responsibility can be delegated to the medical staff, but the final accountability resides with the hospital and its governing board. Although subsequent cases have modified and refined this landmark ruling, it has resulted in a fundamental change in the behavior of hospital administrators and trustees toward physicians in regard to establishing institutional accountability for physician behavior. It has provided administrators and trustees with a degree of legal clout.

The economic forces are twofold. First is the general concern about the inflationary economy, which has made it more costly for many organizations to function. Second, and more specifically, has been the concern over the continued above-average increases in the cost of medical care and hospital services in particular. This has led to a number of regulatory cost containment initiatives, including health systems agencies (HSAs); the PSROs; and, in a number of states, hospital rate review commissions. In addition, some states have experimented with hospital reimbursement based on comparable diagnostic case mix. It is beyond the purview of this paper to address the efficacy of these approaches to cost containment, but there is no question that hospitals have been operating in a environment of increasingly constrained resources, particularly over the past five years. From the perspective of hospital decision making, the most important consequence has been that administrators have gained power and influence in their negotiations with physicians to contain costs. Administrators may not agree with the regulations, but they can use them as an "external scapegoat" for promoting more efficient decision making by physicians in the use of hospital resources. In brief, hospitals and hospital administrators have been provided with greater economic clout.

The societal factors are complex but involve three primary considerations: (1) the demythification of the professions, including medicine; (2) the development of lifestyle alternatives emphasizing disease prevention, health promotion, and self-care; and (3) the rise of professionally trained health care managers. As access to higher education, particularly graduate education, has increased, some of the idealized self-images of the professions have been exposed to wider scrutiny. Furthermore, as society's problems have become more complex and intractable, the limitations of the professions to deal with them have become more obvious. Medicine has become a part of this process. Although still among the highest-rated professions, it no longer enjoys the same unquestioned respect and trust that it did 20 to 30 years ago. This is particularly true in areas outside its own domain of technical competence.

Even within medicine's domain of competence or its "functional specificity,"[10] more people are recognizing its limitations.[11] It is becoming increasingly recognized that good health is more strongly associated with genetics; environment; and lifestyle factors of diet, exercise, and management of stress than with the provision of medical services. Although clearly there are many exceptions (e.g., certain immunizations and some surgical procedures and drugs that promote both the quality and length of life), many Americans no longer see as close an association between good medical care and a healthy life as was true in the past. The above two events, the demythification of the medical profession and the development of alternative approaches to a healthy life, have created a new social context within which hospitals and physicians must operate. Both are subject to intense public scrutiny and an increased degree of "healthy skepticism" regarding their ability to provide services in a cost-effective fashion. In brief, a societal incentive has been provided to hospitals and physicians to work more cooperatively in meeting the changing needs and expectations of a more sophisticated and discriminating public.

To the above may be added the increase in the number of professionally trained health care managers. With greater training in financial management, quantitative methods, organizational behavior, marketing, and interpersonal relations, these managers have gained increased respect and trust from both hospital trustees and physicians. Seeing the need for increased clinical input into hospital decision making, these managers may also feel less threatened by such involvement and may be more willing to work with physicians in exerting joint leadership.

The legal clout, economic clout, and societal incentive described above are altering the relative balance of power between hospitals and physicians. It is no longer in the physician's economic interest to stand aloof from the process, and the hospital stands to gain by bringing resources more under the control of the organization—although at the "price" of greater physician involvement in hospital-wide decision making.

Strain Among Decision Makers and Between the Two Models

There are inherent strains between the needs of organizations and the needs of the professionals associated with them. These strains particularly affect hospital/physician relationships and the two models of decision making described above. Some of the more important strains are summarized in Table 4 and briefly noted below.

First, organizations have a high need for predictability in order to achieve their goals. In contrast, professionals have a high need for freedom to operate in the face of uncertainty. This is most widely recognized in the "exceptional cases" syndrome whereby health care professionals, physicians in particular, can assert that a given case is an "emergency" and thereby set aside the usual rules and regulations.

The organization also has a high need for goal commitment, particularly in regard to survival and effectiveness. Professionals, on the other hand, have a high need for professional goal commitment, which

TABLE 4   Inherent Strains Between Organizational and Professional Needs

ORGANIZATIONAL NEEDS	PROFESSIONALS' NEEDS
1. Predictability.	1. Freedom to operate in the face of uncertainty; the "exceptional case" syndrome.
2. Commitment to organizational goals—maintenance of the organization.	2. Commitment to the goals of one's profession and peers; more narrowly focused than the organization's goals.
3. Coordination/integration across tasks, services, and departments.	3. Freedom to function within specialized interest areas; "loose" coordination that does not interfere with one's professional work.
4. Control and feedback to ensure public accountability.	4. Emphasis on individual accountability to patients and professional peers.
5. Diffuse division of labor (specialization) to accomplish organizational-relevant tasks.	5. Fairly rigid specialization to accomplish individual-specific tasks.

SOURCE: Shortell, S. M. "Theory Z: Implications and Relevance for Health Care Management." *Health Care Management Review* 7 (Fall 1982), p. 11.

is less widely focused than organizational goals and tends to be centered more on individual patient treatment.

Organizations also have a high need for coordination and integration across tasks, services, and departments. In contrast, professionals have a high need for freedom to function within specialized interests. As Weisbord notes: "In medicine, professionals believe in their bones that procedures and organizational needs for . . . survival will be inimical to theirs."[12]

Organizations have a high need for control and feedback, particularly concerning their public accountability. In contrast, professionals have a high need for individual accountability to patients and to professional peers.

Finally, organizations have a relatively high need for specialization to accomplish tasks. Professionals also have a high need for specialization but not necessarily in a manner compatible with the needs of the organization.

Overall, the organization's needs are largely macro in nature, reflecting the overall goals of the organization and the relationship of the organization to its larger environment. At the same time the organization's needs are primarily local in the sense that the commitment is to the organization, with professionals viewed as a vehicle for achievement of the organization's goals. In contrast, health care professionals are largely concerned with micro issues centered on individual patient care but with a cosmopolitan orientation characterized by a commitment to professional growth in the development of one's speciality. In brief, the organization is seen as the vehicle for the achievement of professional goals.

These are some of the fundamental differences that must be taken into account and managed whether one adopts a dual authority or shared authority decision-making model. In general, the above differences tend to reinforce the dual authority model and make it more difficult to bring about a shared model.

Types of Physician Decision-Making Involvement

Decision-making involvement takes two primary forms: formal and informal. The principal modes of formal physician involvement in hospital decision making are participation in meetings of the board of trustees and in the committee structure of the board, the administration, and the medical staff itself and in hospital/physician compensation arrangements whereby the physician is economically tied to the hospital's welfare.

The primary methods of informal involvement include interaction among administrators, trustees, medical staff members, and nurses along with informal ad hoc group discussion of issues as they arise. In general, the degree of formalization of the decision-making process increases with hospital size and complexity, although informal elements are always present. Also, in general, routine decisions such as changing inventory levels or adding a new staff member are made by individuals in the appropriate position or processed through the appropriate formal committee. Nonroutine decisions such as adding or dropping a major program usually are first discussed in informal ad hoc discussion groups, involving those with the most at stake. Only after some closure or at least clarification of the issue has been obtained will it be brought before appropriate committees for further discussion and a decision. In many cases the decision will have been made already, and the committee will simply rubber stamp it. In these nonroutine decisions it is often difficult to identify a single, clear-cut decision maker, and, indeed, the decisions themselves may not be clearly identifiable acts.[13]

Some systematic descriptive information exists on the degree of physician participation in hospital governing bodies and committees and on the percentage of hospital-compensated physicians. These data indicate that 42 percent of hospitals have one or more active staff physicians as voting members of their governing boards.[14] Twenty-six percent of hospitals have physicians as members of the executive committee of the governing board, the group that usually conducts much of the board's business. The percentage of board members who are physicians is generally not related to bed size nor teaching status but is strongly related to ownership. Specifically, between 52 and 64 percent of for-profit hospital board members are physicians compared with approximately 11 to 26 percent for voluntary hospitals.[15] Approximately 60 percent of for-profit hospitals have boards on which physicians are in the majority.[16] At the same time, for-profit hospitals have relatively little physician involvement in committees other than board activities. This suggests that in for-profit hospitals physician involvement in decision making in centered primarily in the governance activities of the institution rather than in the committee structure per se.[17] Voluntary hospitals exhibit an opposite pattern, having greater physician participation in committees but less participation in governing board activities.

It is important to note, however, that physician involvement in hospital governing board activities says nothing about the degree of influence that governing boards exert over hospital policy and operation. In this regard there may be as much or more variability among investor-owned hospitals and among voluntary hospitals than between the two types. The Hospital Corporation of America (HCA), for example, operates on a strongly decentralized basis in which local hospital governing boards maintain some degree of discretion and influence, although accountability remains centralized. In contrast, Humana, Inc., operates on a highly centralized basis with more operating decisions made at the corporate office level and less autonomy provided to individual hospitals. The relative influence of hospital governing boards in investor-owned hospitals, freestanding voluntary hospitals, and voluntary multi-unit systems is an important issue for further investigation. For example, it is commonly believed that the influence of individual hospital boards is diminished in multi-unit systems, whether investor-owned or voluntary. But no systematic information is available to indicate the extent to which this is true or in what specific areas or types of decision making such differences may exist.

Overall, hospitals have approximately 4 medical staff committees per 100 beds.[18] Two key committees are the joint conference committee, made up of trustee, hospital administration, and medical staff leaders, and the medical staff executive committee itself. Although all accredited hospitals are required to have these two committees, their actual influence and practice varies widely. Other common committees are medical audit, utilization review, credentials, and the infection committee. The average number of committee members is 6, and the committees meet an average of 11 times per year. Approximately one-third of the medical staff committees have a nonphysician, usually an administrator or a nurse, with voting representation. For 58 percent of the committees the members are appointed either by the medical staff president, the hospital administrator, or by both acting jointly, rather than being elected by the staff.

In regard to physician compensation arrangements, nationally 25 percent of active staff physicians have some type of hospital financial arrangement, either part time or full time.[19] Twenty-eight percent of department chiefs are on contract. Of all active staff with a contract, 23 percent are salaried. Arrangements whereby physicians are compensated by hospitals are more often found in teaching hospitals than in nonteaching hospitals.[20] They also are more common in for-profit hospitals than in voluntary hospitals.[21]

Systematic longitudinal data are not available, but a general reading of the literature and conversations with hospital administrators and medical staffs suggest that physician involvement in governing board activities, participation in committees, and hospital-based compensation arrangements is growing. For example, over the past five years a number of hospitals have added cost containment committees, medical equipment purchase committees, and strategic long-range planning committees, all with physician participation. Thus, there appears to be a growing trend toward the shared authority model of decision making described earlier or at least deliberate attempts to blur the clear demarcation suggested by the dual authority model. Some of the effects of these changes on the cost and quality of patient care are examined below.

Hospital/Physician Decision Making and the Cost and Quality of Care

The issue of hospital/physician decision making is important primarily as it affects the delivery of patient care services. The relevant question is whether certain patterns of decision making are associated with improvements in the cost-effectiveness of the care delivered. Present research does not provide a clear-cut answer in terms of cause and effect, but the majority of the existing evidence suggests consistent associations between greater physician involvement in hospital decision making and lower costs. Existing research also suggests consistent associations between greater physician participation and higher quality of care. There is little evidence that costs can be contained only at the expense of lowering the quality of care. If anything, the evidence suggests that efforts to contain costs can be associated with improvements in the quality of care.

It is important to note that the research on the relationship between physician involvement in hospital decision making and the cost and quality of care has almost all been conducted in voluntary hospitals. Thus, little is known about this relationship in for-profit hospitals. This is another area for future research.

Evidence Regarding Costs

A number of studies have examined the relationship between various aspects of physician involvement in hospital decision making and cost of care.[22] These studies generally indicate that the more aware physicians are of the organization's performance and the greater the number of scheduled meetings between such key clinical and patient care departments as radiology, laboratory, and nursing service, the lower the costs will be in specific medical support departments. Some evidence also suggests that for-profit hospitals have a higher ratio of nurses and physicians to support personnel, which in turn is more strongly associated with occupancy rates in for-profit hospitals than in not-for-profit hospitals.[23] This may be due to the stronger economic orientation of the for-profit hospital, although in the current climate of economic constraint, not-for-profit hospitals also have a high need for surplus revenues. Thus, differences in economic orientation of for-profit versus not-for-profit hospitals may be narrowing.

The percentage of hospital-based physicians on contract also has been found to be positively associated with lower costs per admission, and physician presence on the executive committee of the governing board also is associated with lower costs per admission.[24]

Evidence Regarding Quality

A number of investigators have examined how the relationship between physicians and hospitals may affect the quality of patient care.[25] In general, these studies suggest that greater physician participation in hospital decision making is positively associated with higher quality of care, as measured by such indicators as severity-adjusted death rates and postsurgical complication rates. There is also evidence that the greater the hospital administrators' ability to influence decisions within their domain, the higher the quality of care.[26] Others have found positive relationships between quality of care and more highly structured medical staffs, as measured by appointment procedures, number of control committees, and percentage of physicians on contract.[27] Morlock et al. also found evidence of a strong relationship between hospital trustee involvement in hospital decision making and the quality of care.[28] In their study, hospitals with influential trustees were much more likely to have medical staff committees that met frequently and were more likely to produce frequent internal monitoring reports on quality of care statistics.

Evidence Regarding Possible Trade-Offs Between Cost and Quality

A major issue in physician/hospital decision making is the extent to which control of costs or improved efficiency can be achieved only at the expense of the quality of care. Most of the studies to date, however, suggest that efforts at containing costs are positively associated with quality. For example, a study of Chicago-area hospitals found that the more efficient hospitals, as measured by lower costs and lower man-hours per standardized unit of output, also provided higher-quality care, as evaluated by outside experts and as indicated by accreditation and severity-adjusted death rates.[29] A study of hospitals in Massa-

chusetts revealed that higher cost per case was associated with higher
medical/surgical death rates, even when differences in case mix were
taken into account.[30] Other studies have generally found similar results.[31] However, Flood et al. found that hospitals that provide a greater
number of certain specific medical services that increase cost also had
better than expected patient care outcomes.[32] In this study the relationship between overall cost and measures of quality of care was not
examined.

It is important to note that the above results are preliminary and
suggestive at best, and they must be viewed with caution. Nonetheless,
existing evidence offers little support for the argument or expectation
that efficiency or cost containment goals are inherently incompatible
with effectiveness or quality of care. It may be that greater physician
involvement in hospital-wide administrative decision making facilitates cost containment decisions that protect or even enhance the
quality of care provided. For example, changes to improve the turn-
around time for laboratory tests not only improve hospital efficiency
but may also improve quality of care by expediting the physician's
diagnostic and treatment plans for the patient. Clearly, this is a major
area for future research and public policy development. The effects of
physician involvement in hospital-wide decision making on the overall
use of hospital services is another important area for further investigation.

Future Issues

It should be evident from the above discussion that physician involvement in hospital decision making is in flux. As indicated, this is primarily due to changes in the external environment of health care
delivery, which is causing physicians and hospitals to view themselves
and each other in a different light. As a clue to the future it is useful
to consider the changing context of both clinical decision making and
institutional decision making. The possible demise of the traditional
voluntary medical staff organization can be foreseen. It then becomes
possible to consider the factors that either promote or constrain the
movement toward more shared, collaborative decision-making models.

The Changing Context of Clinical Decision Making

Pellegrino has commented that:

The process of making clinical decisions is the balance wheel of hospital operation.
It is central to all the patient-oriented functions of the hospital, and it has remote
effects on all major elements of hospital organization—the patient, the health

care professional, administrators, trustees, and the community. It is also the process least accessible to organizational control, the most in need of freedom, and yet the most potent of hospital processes for good and evil. The clinical decision is the most zealously guarded of the physician's prerogatives and at the same time the most in need of some kind of surveillance for individual and public good. It is, moreover, the most difficult process to evaluate in a definitive way.[33]

Five factors are redefining the context of clinical decision making: (1) the realization that resources are scarce—a "logic of scarcity," (2) the continued impact of new technology, (3) changes in the mix of diseases being seen, (4) the increased institutionalization of all aspects of medical care, and (5) the effects of the consumer movement.

The concern over the cost of health care has resulted in a logic of scarcity that is beginning to permeate medical practice. There exists a subtle and still-developing change from the norm of "doing everything possible for the patient at all costs" to one of "doing only those things that might reasonably yield positive outcomes" and choosing the most cost-effective ways of doing those procedures. In the extreme this is resulting in the use of cost-benefit assessments in making decisions to treat some patients and not others. This is a profound and very important change. Never before has such a logic been a part of the "micro-level" of the health care system, the level of individual clinical decision making.

Continued advances in technology require continual rethinking of diagnostic and treatment protocols and clinical decision-making rules. This increases the rate of change and uncertainty, which in turn leads to greater specialization of function and greater competition among specialties. One example is the recent dispute among pathologists, radiologists, and internists over developments in nuclear medicine. Specifically, pathologists claim they have the facilities, space, and personnel to handle large-scale procedures; radiologists maintain they have the techniques; and internists, of course, note that they have the patients. A partial solution appears to have been worked out in the development of a conjoint board that is sponsored by all three specialties and that allows access to certification in nuclear medicine from each of them.

There have also been appreciable changes in the mix of diseases being seen—specifically in the chronic, complex conditions associated with aging. One implication of this change is that teams of different kinds of specialists and providers are needed to provide effective care. This further complicates the clinical decision-making process and raises a number of issues involving who should be the team leader and who should assume various roles and responsibilities.

As previously noted, medical care is increasingly an organizational process, subject to organizational forms of social control. The *Darling* decision, which held hospitals and their governing boards ultimately responsible for quality of care, helped give rise to PSROs and related institutionalized forms of review.

Finally, there is continued interest by the public in having more control over their own lives, and, as previously noted, this has affected the health care professions. The public has a desire to know more and to be given more choices, including the choice not to seek or comply with medical advice. Manifestations are emerging both in collective bodies such as health planning agencies and at the level of the individual provider-patient relationship. As such, they have affected clinical decision making, if only as a sensitizing factor that further complicates the decision-making process.

The effect of these five factors has been to transform the context in which clinical decisions are made. In brief, such decisions are no longer within the exclusive domain of the medical profession; the boundaries have become more permeable, allowing participation by other providers, health care organizations, regulatory groups, consumers, and others. The issue is whether the continued prevalence of dual authority decision-making structures or the continuing emergence of shared decision-making authority structures provides a better forum for dealing with the increased complexity and diffuseness of clinical decision making.

The Changing Context of Institutional Decision Making

Not only are hospitals under increased public scrutiny because of the continuing rise in costs, but it also seems likely that hospitals will remain under such scrutiny permanently. This is not only because of the continued concern regarding the cost-effectiveness of patient care but also because hospitals, individually and collectively, have taken on more characteristics of industrial enterprises central to the American economy. Many individual hospitals are joining multi-unit systems to gain greater economic and political clout. Approximately 26 percent of all hospitals belong to a multi-unit system now, and estimates suggest that close to 80 percent may belong to such systems by 1990.[34] Even among individual hospitals there has been growth in professional managerial staff specialists, marketing specialists, long-range planning departments, and health services research units.

Regulation of capital and operating expenses plus an inflationary economy have forced hospitals to compete more with each other for patients, physicians, and nurses. In many areas of the country, voluntary hospitals are competing directly with investor-owned hospitals, and teaching hospitals are competing with nonteaching hospitals. The result is that voluntary and investor-owned hospitals are becoming more alike, ironically as a result of trying to differentiate their services in an attempt to find new markets for growth. Thus, some voluntary hospitals are entering into management contract relationships with other voluntary hospitals and are forming systems that are similar to those of investor-owned hospitals, and some investor-owned hospitals are beginning to offer outreach and satellite services similar to those offered by voluntary hospitals. Teaching hospitals are becoming more like their community hospital counterparts in offering more general primary care services and community outreach services, and community hospitals are striving to expand their markets by adding the more sophisticated technology found in teaching hospitals.

American hospitals are no longer a cottage industry; they are part of an industry that is becoming more highly concentrated, more competitive, and more heavily interdependent with other organizations. It is also an industry that is extremely vulnerable to economic, regulatory, and technological changes. As such, decision making, particularly at the upper policymaking levels of the organization, has become a very complex and difficult process. The number of inspirational decisions relative to computational decisions has increased. There is an increased need to turn more of these inspirational decisions into judgmental or compromise decisions.

There also is a greater need for clinical participation in the administrative decision-making process and consideration of more administrative and economic matters in the clinical decision-making process. The following question may be raised: Is the current relationship of physicians to hospitals, in the form of the voluntary medical staff, able to meet the challenge of the new decision-making environment? In brief, is the voluntary medical staff organization structure rapidly becoming an anachronism?

The Demise of the Voluntary Medical Staff

Fundamental changes in the structure of medical staff organization may be taking place already. A growing number of physicians are affiliating with hospitals as a cost-effective way of starting practices, a growing number of speciality-trained physicians are contracting with one or more hospitals to deliver secondary and tertiary care services, and a growing number of hospital medical staffs are entering into HMO arrangements of various forms.[35] As the predicted physician surplus materializes over the next decade, competition among physicians will grow, and many will look to the above kinds of arrangements to gain competitive advantages. But what effect will these trends have on physician/hospital decision-making relationships? Although it is safe to say that the dual authority model will continue to prevail in most settings, it is likely that shifts toward more shared models will become more prevalent, depending on a number of factors, highlighted below, that may facilitate or constrain such a movement.

Factors Promoting or Impeding Shared Decision-Making Models

Expectations of more shared decision making between physicians and hospitals can be based on several arguments. The first is that the physician surplus will make physicians more dependent on hospitals for privileges and services to build and maintain their practices; thus, their economic well-being will become more closely identified with that of the hospital. This will provide a stimulus for more joint physician/hospital involvement in decision making. Second, as regulation (at any governmental level) continues, physicians and hospitals may perceive increased incentives to unite against the "common enemy." Consistent with the "capture" theory of regulation (whereby the industry itself desires the regulation so as to protect its own interest), physicians and hospitals will work together to make sure their mutual interests are protected. Hospital reimbursement based on case mix also may require more collaborative decision making as such reimbursement requires administrative and cost data to be integrated with clinical data.

Third, as physicians become more closely aligned to hospitals, they may demand greater participation in hospital-wide decision making than they currently have through traditional medical staff organization channels. In brief, they may seek to have greater influence with an organization that is gaining greater importance in their professional lives.

Finally, shared decision-making models may be facilitated by more sophisticated and enlightened physicians and professionally trained hospital administrators. More physicians are being exposed to the importance of cost-effective medical care and associated cost-effectiveness and cost-benefit methodologies. Some, such as graduates of the Robert Wood Johnson Foundation's Clinical Scholars Program, have received broad exposure to health services and health policy issues. Thus, there may be emerging a new cadre of medical leadership with a broader understanding of the hospital both as an economic and a social institution, which overrides the notion of the hospital as simply the "doctor's workshop." As noted by the Hospital Association of Pennsylvania:

> The hospital-medical staff relationship is currently the weakest link in the hospital corporate management structure. It is this weakness, together with the rising cost issue, which will force a new relationship between physicians and hospitals in the very near future.
>
> Joint decision-making involving medical staffs will need to be developed to gain their participation in an acceptance of change in institutional procedures.[36]

On the other hand, several factors could impede the development of shared decision-making models. First, increased physician competition, resulting from the developing surplus of physicians, could result in more physicians offering services in direct competition with hospitals. Emerging examples include emergency care, sports medicine, and health promotion. Under increasing competition, primary care physicians in particular may seek to develop special services. Whether they choose to compete directly with hospitals will depend on a number of local market factors and customs, including the power of local hospitals, the demographic composition of the community, and the organization of the medical practice community itself. For example, it would be difficult for a new solo practitioner to compete with a hospital, but it would be easier if new physicians could join well-established group practices and develop new programs and services from that base.

A second factor that may cause physicians to keep an arm's-length relationship with hospitals is the physician's desire to escape the regulation and reimbursement controls imposed on hospitals. If physicians see little opportunity to change the regulatory or payment climate by working with hospitals, some will move to distance themselves from its consequences by becoming as autonomous as possible. This will have essentially the same effect as noted above in regard to competition, i.e., the provision of more services in the physician's offices. For such services as radiology and pathology this has already resulted in the purchase of more sophisticated equipment for physician's offices (e.g., computed tomographic scanners), as opposed to locating them in the hospital.

A third deterrent to the development of more shared decision making models may be the unwillingness of hospital administrators to open up the decision-making process to physicians. This is likely to be a significant issue in many areas and is understandable given the historical evolution of administrator-physician relationships in U.S.

hospitals. Essentially, administrators have used informal and persuasive skills (in addition to the legitimate authority derived from their positions) to gain influence over medical staffs. In particular, they have used their role as intermediary between the medical staff and the board of trustees to control communication and information flow and thus to keep some control over the medical staff's influence on the board. The idea of involving physicians more systematically in hospital-wide policymaking presents a major challenge for administrators and physicians alike.

Summary

This paper has attempted to capture some of the complexity and dynamics of changing physician/hospital decision-making relationships. A typology and a number of examples of physician/hospital decision making were developed to provide a framework for considering current developments. Some differences were suggested in decision-making strategies by hospital ownership and whether the hospital belonged to a multi-unit system. Two major models of physician/hospital relationships were described—the dual authority model and the shared authority model. The implications of each of these along with the forces influencing their continued development were examined. Evidence regarding the association of more shared decision-making models and the cost and quality of care was summarized. A number of issues pertaining to the changing context of clinical and institutional decision making were presented, suggesting that some fundamental changes may take place in the structure of hospital medical staffs.

These points have a number of possible implications for for-profit hospitals. First, they are likely to continue to be somewhat more selective than voluntary hospitals in their choice of services to offer the community. Specifically, they will tend to offer services that enhance the return on the overall portfolio or mix of services provided. Because of the greater involvement of physicians in hospital governance, for-profit hospitals may be more reluctant to compete directly with their medical staffs and more likely to offer services that are complementary to rather than substitutable for physician services in the community.

Second, for-profit hospitals, particularly those owned by investor-owned chains, may be better able than voluntary hospitals to deal with "compromise" or "judgmental" decisions. This is because they have a more clearly defined and homogenous group of constituents (stockholders) and generally more overall centralized direction from the corporate headquarters office. As a result, preferences regarding desired outcomes may be more clear. Investor-owned hospitals may, therefore, be more able to make rapid adjustment to external changes (e.g., changes in third-party reimbursement or changes in competition) than most voluntary hospitals can.

Third, because the interests of physicians and the hospital may be more closely aligned in for-profit hospitals, the dual authority model of decision making is less problematic. Perhaps the lesser degree of physician involvement in daily committee work that characterizes for-profit hospitals reflects a higher degree of agreement on a more homogenous and targeted set of goals and greater physician involvement in the governance process. In contrast, voluntary hospitals deal with the issues created by the dual authority model through a rather elaborate system of committees attempting to achieve increased physician participation and involvement. Although both types of hospitals may be shifting toward a more shared authority model, investor-owned hospitals may be able to make the adjustment more quickly and easily because of the greater degree of agreement on overall goals and the history of physician involvement in decision making at the governance level of the organization.

But it is also important to note that the above differences and their implications may be attenuated by some growing similarities between for-profit and voluntary hospitals in their economic orientations. Under pressures for cost containment, plus increased competition, voluntary hospitals have had to give more concerted thought both to their short-run operational needs and to longer-run capital formation requirements. A number of voluntary hospitals have corporately reorganized, in many instances creating for-profit subsidiaries to expand the hospital's sources of revenue. Some of the above differences may also be attenuated by the continued growth of multi-unit systems among not-for-profit hospitals. Through their corporate office expertise and structure, such systems may be able to offer the same kinds of advantages as the investor-owned systems. In brief, although important differences still exist between the mission, philosophy, structure, and decision making of for-profit and not-for-profit hospitals, forces are currently in motion that over time may diminish some of these differences.

References and Notes

1. Thompson, J. D. *Organizations in Action*. New York: McGraw-Hill, 1967.
2. Shortell, S. M., T. Wickizer, J. Wheeler et al. *Hospital Sponsored Primary Care:*

100 STEPHEN M. SHORTELL

3. Harris, J. E. "The Internal Organization of Hospitals: Some Economic Implications." *Bell Journal of Economics* 8 (1978), p. 479

4. Pauly, M. V., and M. Redisch. "The Not-for-Profit Hospital as Physician's Cooperative." *The American Economic Review* 63 (March 1973), pp. 87-100.

5. Harris, op. cit., pp. 467-482.

6. Smith, H. L. "Two Lines of Authority Are One Too Many." *Modern Hospital* 84 (March 1955), pp. 59-64.

7. Harris, op. cit., p. 477.

8. Scott, W. R. "Managing Professional Work: Three Models of Control for Health Organizations." *Health Services Research* 17 (Fall 1982), pp. 213-240.

9. *Darling* v. *Charleston Community Memorial Hospital*, 211 N.E. Second 253 (1965).

10. Parsons, T. *The Social System.* Glencoe, Ill.: Free Press, 1956.

11. Carlson, R. J. *The End of Medicine.* New York: John Wiley & Sons, 1975.

12. Weisbord, M. R. "Why Organization Development Hasn't Worked (So Far) in Academic Medical Centers." *Health Care Management Review* 1 (Spring 1976), p. 18.

13. Allison, R. F., and J. W. Dalston. "Governance of University-Owned Teaching Hospitals." *Inquiry* 19 (Spring 1982), pp. 3-17.

14. Shortell, S. M., and T. Getzen. "Measuring Hospital Medical Staff Organization and Structures." *Health Services Research* 14 (Summer 1979), pp. 97-110.

15. Sloan, F. A. "The Internal Organization of Hospitals: A Descriptive Study." *Health Services Research* 15 (Fall 1980), pp. 294-230.

16. Ibid.

17. Shortell, S. M., and C. Evashwick. "The Structural Configuration of U.S. Hospital Medical Staffs." *Medical Care* 19 (April 1981), pp. 419-430.

18. Sloan, op. cit.

19. Bidece, L., and D. Danais. *Physician Characteristics and Distribution in the United States—1981.* Chicago: Division of Survey and Data Resources, American Medical Association, 1982.

20. Sloan, op. cit.

21. Shortell and Evashwick, op. cit.

22. Neuhauser, D. *The Relationship Between Administrative Practices and Hospital Performance.* Chicago: Center for Health Administration Studies, University of Chicago, Research Series #28, 1971; Shortell, S. M., S. W. Becker, and D. Neuhauser. "The Effects of Management Practices on Hospital Efficiency and Quality of Care." *Organizational Research in Hospitals: An Inquiry Monograph*, S. M. Shortell and M. Brown, eds. Chicago: Blue Cross Association, 1976, pp. 90-106; Rushing, W. "Differences in Profit and Nonprofit Organizations: A Study of Effectiveness and Efficiency in General Short-Stay Hospitals." *Administrative Science Quarterly* 19 (December 1974), pp. 473-484; Pauly, M. "Medical Staff Characteristics and Hospital Costs." *Journal of Human Resources*, Supplement 13 (1978), p. 77; Sloan, F., and E. Becker. "International Organization of Hospitals and Hospital Costs." *Inquiry* 18 (Fall 1981), pp. 224-239.

23. Rushing, op. cit.

24. Pauly, op. cit.

25. Neuhauser, op. cit.; Shortell, Becker, and Neuhauser, op. cit.; Flood, A., and W. R. Scott. "Professional Power and Professional Effectiveness: The Power of the Surgical Staff and the Quality of Surgical Care in Hospitals." *Journal of Health and Social Behavior* 19 (September 1978), p. 240; Roemer, M., and J. Friedman. *Doctors in Hospitals: Medical Staff Organization and Hospital Performance.* Baltimore: Johns Hopkins University Press, 1971; Shortell, S. M., and J. P. LoGerfo. "Hospital Medical Staff Organization and Quality of Care: Results for Myocardial Infarction and Appendectomy." *Medical Care* 19 (October 1981), pp. 1041-1056; Rhee, S. "Relative Importance of Physician's Personal and Situational Characteristics for the Quality of Patient Care." *Journal of Health and Social Behavior* 18

(March 1977), pp. 10-15; Morlock, L., C. Nathanson, D. N. Schumacher, and S. D. Horn. "Decision-Making Patterns and Hospital Performance: Relationships Between Case Mix Adjusted Mortality Rates and the Influence of Trustee, Administrators, and Medical Staff in Seventeen Acute Care General Hospitals." *Medical Care*, in press; Holland, P. P., A. Konick, W. Buffum et al. "Institutional Structure and Resident Outcome." *Journal of Health and Social Behavior* 22 (December 1981), pp. 433-444.

26. Flood and Scott, op. cit.

27. Roemer and Friedman, op. cit.

28. Morlock et al., op. cit.

29. Neuhauser, op. cit.

30. Shortell, Becker, and Neuhauser, op. cit.

31. Longest, B. B. "An Empirical Analysis of the Quality-Cost Relationship." *Hospital and Health Services Administration* 23 (Fall 1978), pp. 20-35; Schulz, R. I., J. R. Greenley, and R. W. Peterson. "Management, Cost and Quality in Hospitals." *Medical Care*, in press.

32. Flood, A. B., W. Ewy, and W. R. Scott et al. "The Relationship Between Intensity and Duration of Medical Services and Outcomes for Hospitalized Patients." *Medical Care* 17 (1979), pp. 1088-1102.

33. Pellegrino, E. D. "The Changing Matrix of Clinical Decision-Making in the Hospital." In *Organizational Research in Health Institutions*, B. S. Georgopoulos, ed. Ann Arbor: University of Michigan Press Institute for Survey Research, 1972, p. 301.

34. Brown, M. "Multi-Hospital Systems: Trends, Issues, and Prospects." In *Multi-Hospital Systems: Policy Issues for the Future*, G. Bisbee, Jr., ed. Chicago: The Hospital Research Educational Trust, 1981, pp. 3-21.

35. Morrisey, M. "A Description of Hospital-HMO Affiliations." Paper presented at the American Public Health Association Meetings, Montreal, Quebec, Canada, November 1982.

36. Pennsylvania Hospital Association. *Environmental Assessment.* Hospital Industry and Hospital Association of Pennsylvania, Camp Hill, Pennsylvania, February 1981, p. 35.

Economic Incentives and Clinical Decisions

Harold S. Luft

The recent growth of for-profit activities in medical care has led to concern about the growth of a "new medical-industrial complex" (Relman, 1980; see also Caper, 1982; Saward and Sorensen, 1982). These concerns range from the fear that such enterprises will skim off all the profitable patients and leave the voluntary and public sectors with mounting bad debts to the fear that patients will lose their trust in the medical profession. There is also an emerging controversy over the possibility that for-profit health care entails some economic incentives that may affect day-to-day clinical decisions. Will physicians who own hospitals, laboratories, or other for-profit enterprises, or who work for a national chain of hospitals or urgent care clinics, practice differently from those who do not? These concerns are based on a more general question of the extent to which economic incentives affect physicians' decisions about patient care.

This paper is about clinical or patient care decisions, such as whether to order an X-ray for an ankle injury, rather than about production decisions, such as whether needed equipment should be leased or purchased. No one seems to question the notion that economic factors do (and probably should) influence production decisions, nor do people

I am indebted to Bradford Gray, Susan Maerki, Victor Rodwin, Anne Scitovsky, Jonathan Showstack, Joan Trauner, and anonymous referees for their helpful comments on earlier drafts.

seem very concerned about the propriety of for-profit enterprises in this arena. Profit incentives seem to be acceptable as long as they are limited to how certain services are provided and as long as the professionals who order the services and evaluate their quality are insulated from the proprietary system. Such incentives are being questioned, however, when they potentially affect physicians who decide what services are needed and whether the care delivered is of appropriate quality.

To help set the stage for a larger investigation of ethical and professional concerns about physician involvement in for-profit enterprises in health care, this paper addresses a relatively simple question: In the current environment, to what extent do economic or financial incentives influence physicians' clinical or patient care decisions?

Unfortunately, physicians and economists offer markedly different answers to the question. Unlike the situation of the 8-ounce glass containing 4 ounces of water, the responses reflect more than semantics. Physicians typically argue that such incentives have little influence, except in a few obvious and distressing cases, such as fee splitting and kickbacks and, furthermore, that economic incentives should have no place in clinical decisions. Economists maintain the opposite view: Such incentives are ubiquitous and have a major influence. Some economists would argue that expanding incentives and freeing physicians to use them would cure the ills of the medical care sector. For instance, some economists would like to see the physician more free to serve as the patient's agent, taking into account both the medical and economic consequences of alternative clinical decisions. Other economists think that a greater role of economic incentives could exacerbate current problems.

Although the physicians' and economists' positions have been overdrawn for the sake of exposition, the perceptions are so divergent that an examination of the models of clinical decision making used by the physician and the economist is warranted. The differences in these models partially explain why the answers to the simple question of the influence of economic incentives are so divergent. The following section reviews the evidence on the effects of economic incentives on physician behavior, prefaced by a discussion of what is considered acceptable evidence by physicians and economists. The third section offers a synthesis of the two views, suggesting how economic incentives can have an important role in decision making despite being invisible to the clinician. A final section provides a brief summary and conclusions.

Models of Clinical Decision Making

The usual medical model of decision making involves a complex and largely intuitive process whereby the physician considers signs, symptoms, and a variety of test results and, based upon scientific knowledge and clinical experience, arrives at a diagnosis and chooses the best treatment (Eddy, 1982). The classic biomedical model presumes a single, potentially identifiable cause of a disease for which there is a single best treatment. Only in recent years has the existence of multiple factors in the causation of disease been recognized by some physicians, along with the recognition that patients may differ in their preferences for or responses to alternative treatments for the same condition (McNeil et al., 1982). The traditional, reductionist single-cause/single-cure model, which long has been at the root of biomedical research and medical education, makes the physician a seeker of truth, who must vigorously resist any deviation from the one right path, for economic or other reasons. This model of behavior has other important implications. The physician is clearly in authority, and the patient must wait to find out the correct course of action. The authority of the physician also implies the responsibility for making the correct diagnosis and for choosing the correct treatment. The implicit responsibility probably contributes to the large volume of malpractice suits.

Diagnosis and treatment decisions often are not clear-cut. However, in practice, many physicians act as if things were clear-cut and develop "standard operating rules" or "clinical policies" that dictate what should be done (Eddy, 1982). These clinical policies may be highly complex, such as: "If signs A, B, and C are present, test X is negative, and there is no history of Y, the appropriate diagnosis is Q and the treatment is R." Furthermore, as will be seen below, experienced physicians may often have different clinical policies. Some physicians, trained in the techniques of decision analysis, argue for the explicit consideration of alternative causes and treatments (McNeil and Adelstein, 1975; Pauker and Kassirer, 1975). Explicit choice making, however, highlights the uncertainties in medicine that the typical physician would often rather ignore. For example, suppose that the available information allows the physician to reduce the problem to the following: "Everything points to the conclusion that the patient has disease Q and the appropriate treatment is R, but there is 1 chance in 100 that it is disease S and the treatment should be T." Most physicians seem to prefer not to deal explicitly with the probabilities and potential outcomes, instead focusing on statements such as: "In my experience the problem seems to be Q, and the correct treatment is R." Because most such clinical policies are based on extensive experience and the decisions generally are accepted by the patients, the results usually are not substantially different from what would be found after a careful decision analysis exercise. And the physician usually sleeps more soundly by ignoring the overwhelming number of implicit probabilities, valuations, and choices that arise each day.

In contrast to medical training, which emphasizes the single best course, economists are trained to believe that there are an infinite number of potential solutions, the selection of which should depend on individual preferences, and that the most efficient allocation of resources will be achieved if everyone pursues his or her own self-interest in a market economy. Furthermore, although physicians have traditionally seen medical problems in terms of immutable laws of chemistry and physics, economists have been expanding the realm of economic analysis, with its emphasis on individual choice and trade-offs, to include politics, the family, and natural selection (Becker, 1981; Wilson, 1978). (The holistic approach in medicine takes a much wider view and recognizes the importance of multiple factors, but it is still far from the mainstream.)

This difference in perspective has clear implications for the way that economic incentives are perceived. Under the traditional physician model the medical problem—and its potential solutions—is dealt with independently from all else. Moreover, although the physician is primarily concerned with the patient's well-being, the evaluation of what is best is usually from the perspective of the physician rather than the patient. The extreme economic view is to include everything in the choice set. For example, Grossman's model of the demand for health views the body as a machine that depreciates yearly until it breaks down and is overhauled (medical intervention) or scrapped (death) and for which preventive maintenance decisions are considered relative to other ways that the owner can spend his or her time and money (Grossman, 1972, 1982). From the economist's perspective, physicians are like auto mechanics, who want to turn every ordinary family car into a luxury machine without considering whether the family would like to spend its time or money on something else, such as a summer vacation.

The analogy to an auto mechanic may distress some physicians, but it incorporates the economist's recognition that many of the technical details of medicine are too complicated for patients to evaluate directly. However, just as few consumers understand the complexities of auto repair, although most can determine whether a car is running better, patients often can evaluate the results of medical care without understanding the disease processes or the therapeutic alternatives. The problem for the patient is to have someone determine what is wrong, to have the treatment choices identified and explained, and to choose the appropriate people to carry out the desired interventions. In this regard the economist views the ideal primary care physician as the patient's agent, providing the relevant information and selecting the appropriate specialists (Feldstein, 1974; Pauly, 1980). (Note the parallel to a trusted mechanic who can diagnose a transmission problem and then identify a competent specialty shop to do the work.) A perfect physician-agent would lead the consumer to precisely the same decision as the consumer would have reached given all of the physician's expertise. This decision may well differ from traditional "best medical practice" because the patient is likely to take into consideration the cost of the services, the time involved in treatment, and other factors not usually involved in choosing the best *medical* outcome.

Although the notion of a perfect agent is a very attractive theoretical concept, there are few perfect agents because of the conventional methods of organizing care and paying physicians. It is often the case that most of the work is in arriving at the diagnosis, so the same physician provides both the diagnosis and the treatment. The dominant mode of payment is fee-for-service, and, more important, fees are heavily weighted toward laboratory tests and diagnostic and therapeutic procedures in contrast to time spent talking with the patient (Schroeder and Showstack, 1978; Showstack et al., 1979). The hypothetical "physician as a perfect agent" would be available and willing to spend time with the patient, investigating the problem, pondering the diagnosis, and calculating the alternatives. The best physician-agent would have no personal economic incentives either to encourage or discourage additional tests and procedures or to prefer one course of treatment over another. In practice, however, except for psychiatrists, fee-for-time arrangements for physicians are uncommon.[1] Furthermore, primary physicians are rarely only counselors, and even the diagnostic function involves many highly profitable tests.

The crucial issue here is not the method of paying the physician—fee-for-service, capitation, or salary—but the linkage between the

[1]Surgeons often charge a fee that includes pre- and postoperative visits, obstetricians have prenatal/maternity packages, and pediatricians sometimes have a single fee for the first year of well-baby care. In most of these cases, however, tests and treatments for complications are handled on a standard fee-for-service basis.

physician as agent and the physician as provider. For instance, many medical school faculty are on a straight salary, yet they know that their department's revenues are dependent on fee-for-service billings and that a revenue shortfall will affect salaries, promotions, and perquisites. Similarly, the medical group in a health maintenance organization (HMO) may receive a capitation payment covering the annual primary care of its enrollees, but if the group orders too much hospital care, its share of the plan's net income will be smaller (Luft, 1981). The incentives to provide services are reversed in some systems—fee-for-service has a bias toward more services while the fixed budget of a HMO sets up a bias toward fewer services—but in each case economic factors are present that could influence clinical decisions. Whether physicians respond to such incentives is another question.

Incentives from the Perspective of the Physician and the Economist

Before reviewing the evidence concerning the role of economic incentives, we must consider what would be recognized as an "influence on clinical decisions." Although the medical literature generally ignores the possibility of such influences, when they are discussed, it seems to be in terms of conscious behavior on the part of the physician. For instance, physicians in prepaid plans have identified as an advantage the fact that all their patients have comprehensive coverage, so the physicians need never be concerned that a proposed treatment would bankrupt the patient (Cook, 1971). Clinicians in fee-for-service practice have mentioned being aware of the gross revenues associated with a procedure while making clinical recommendations (personal communications). Most physicians, however, seem to claim that financial incentives do not influence their patient care decisions.

Economists take a much broader perspective, and, although their language may suggest conscious decision making, they typically care little about what people say they do (or why they do it), focusing their attention instead on behavior. If financial incentives would reward a certain behavior, everything else being equal, then if the behavior is observed, the role of incentives is deemed empirically supported. In this type of analysis the economist typically ignores (or attempts to hold constant statistically) all but the economic variables such as prices and incomes. It is understood that in any particular case, clinical, personal, professional, or other factors may be present and even dominant, but such factors are seen as essentially random. That is, if one considers a large number of cases, these noneconomic factors will cancel out, leaving one able to observe the pattern left by the consistent impact of economic incentives. By contrast, the clinician is trained to focus on precisely those noneconomic factors that the economist dismisses as random and will believe and argue that each case is handled individually, with attention only, or almost only, to the clinical problem. It may be the case that 95 percent of the decision is based on clinical factors and 5 percent on economic factors. The physician will feel that the economic factors are inconsequential, and the economist will respond that if one examines many similar cases, abstracting from the random clinical factors, economics dominates and patterns emerge that cannot be explained by clinical factors.

Yet another difference in approach helps explain the different perceptions of the economist and the physician. The economist tends to be denominator oriented, focusing on the influence of economic variables on various decisions, such as whether individuals experiencing a given set of symptoms decide to see a physician. The physician is typically numerator oriented, focusing on persons who come to the office for care. The physician notes that fees do not influence his or her patients, although the economist responds that fees will determine (at least in part) how many people decide to present themselves as patients.

In most instances the economist attempts to demonstrate a statistically significant effect of an economic variable. The interpretation of such a finding is generally open to question on two grounds. The first is whether the observed *correlation* really implies *causation* or whether other, unobserved factors may be causing the measured relationship. The second is whether the *statistically* significant effect is substantively important. Large samples and sophisticated econometric models often allow very small effects to be measured, but such differences may be of no policy import. From the physician's perspective, subtle tendencies, regardless of the statistical significance or aggregate importance, are inconsequential unless one can identify clear instances in which the economic incentives can be shown to have led to an altered clinical decision. Given the different orientations and tools, the physician's microscope and the economist's telescope, it is not surprising that the two cannot easily agree on what evidence is appropriate. Largely because physician-researchers have not considered the role of incentives a fruitful research area, most of the available evidence uses the economist's approach of searching for tendencies across large numbers of cases. There are, however, a few exceptions that are clinically oriented.

Economic incentives can potentially influence clinical decisions in a wide variety of ways, and it may be useful to consider two broad categories that may bear on subsequent discussions of for-profit enterprise in health care. The first type of incentive or situation involves the physicians' ability to hire other workers (and equipment) and to make more money by owning a larger enterprise. Although the dividing line is not clear, most would perceive a qualitative difference between a physician who hires a nurse practitioner and one who runs a chain of weight reduction clinics. At one end of the spectrum the physician is still primarily a clinician but one who must give some attention to the economic realities of his or her practice. At the other extreme the physician is primarily a business-operator with little day-to-day clinical involvement. The second category of incentives pertains to the way the physician is paid for patient care activities. This includes methods such as fee-for-service, salary, or prepayment with physician responsibility for the costs of prescribed services. It also includes the incentives inherent in each type of payment system, such as relatively higher fees for procedures and tests compared with payment for the physician's time.

Incentives and the Use of Technology

Much of the rapid growth in the use of various medical technologies may stem not just from their clinical efficacy but also from the high returns physicians can get by using such technology. A primary care internist can increase his or her net income by a factor of almost three by prescribing a wide but not unreasonable set of tests (Schroeder and Showstack, 1978). The term *not unreasonable* is a reflection that the use of such tests is so common as to be almost standard practice; yet some clinicians would argue that few of the tests are actually necessary (Griner et al., 1981; Martin, 1982). Some diagnostic technologies, such as endoscopy, have been studied in detail. They are highly profitable, have proliferated rapidly, yet rarely result in a definitive change in treatment outcome (Showstack and Schroeder, 1981). Is this evidence of economic incentives influencing practice patterns? From the economist's perspective, the answer is yes, but the clinician might quickly point out such factors as the low risk of the procedure and the importance of the reassurance it can provide to the patient (and the physician).

A study by Childs and Hunter (1972) of diagnostic X-ray use provides an example of the role of multiple factors in clinical patterns. They examined the use of X-rays for persons under old-age assistance (thus controlling for income and insurance coverage). Patients of physicians who owned their own X-ray equipment (direct providers) were twice as likely to receive an X-ray and were less likely to see a radiologist than were patients of physicians without such equipment. More important, patients of direct providers were much more likely to receive fluoroscopy alone and single-view chest films, procedures generally eschewed by radiologists as providing little useful information. The authors suggest that "the physician with X-ray apparatus, therefore, would be motivated to use that apparatus in order to amortize the capital costs as well as to produce income." They caution, however, that the ease of access may encourage more frequent use. One could argue that physicians who value X-rays more highly (for clinical rather than economic reasons) would be more likely to use them more frequently and therefore purchase the equipment. However, the frequent use of fluoroscopy and single-film studies suggest a lack of clinical sophistication by direct providers.

Technology use in hospitals has grown at a very rapid pace, perhaps more rapidly than in physician's offices, but there are no reliable data for either setting. In the last decade the hospital CT scanner and special care units have become almost ubiquitous, and other "little ticket" technologies have proliferated and added substantially to costs (Fineberg, 1979; Moloney and Rogers, 1979). Tracing the physician's incentives during the inpatient episode is more complex than for outpatient care. In many instances, both the hospital and the physician profit from the test: The hospital charges cover the test itself, such as an EKG, and the physician may charge a separate fee for interpreting the results. Sometimes the physician's fee is influenced by the patient's location; a hospital visit to a patient in intensive care may command a higher fee than a visit on the ward (California Medical Association, 1975). Sometimes the primary physician has no direct economic interest in additional tests, such as CT scans interpreted by radiologists. There can be indirect incentives, however, even without fee splitting. If a test can substitute for the primary physician's time and effort, that time can often be used to advantage elsewhere. Furthermore, if the hospital can profit from increased use of certain procedures, funds may be available to provide the perquisites some physicians find attractive. There is some direct evidence that ancillary costs in proprietary hospitals are significantly higher than in voluntary hospitals (Lewin et al., 1981). In California, ancillary services are used by proprietary hospitals as major profit centers (Blumberg, 1979). What is less clear, however, is whether and how physicians' clinical decisions are altered by proprietary hospitals.

Payment and Practice Setting Incentives

In contrast to the near dearth of studies on incentives and technology, there is considerable evidence concerning the role of direct payment incentives and practice patterns. The clearest distinction is between physicians paid on a fee-for-service basis, in which case there is a clear incentive to do more, and those paid a fixed sum in salary or capitation. Bunker (1970) found that certain discretionary surgical procedures were performed twice as frequently per capita in the United States as in England and Wales. Although the difference in mode of payment—fee-for-service in the United States and salaried in Britain—might explain this difference, the number of surgeons in the United States was also proportionately higher. International comparisons are fraught with difficulty, so studies of different practice settings within the United States may be more conclusive.

In almost all comparisons of persons enrolled in HMOs of the prepaid group practice (PGP) type and those obtaining care in conventional fee-for-service settings, the hospitalization rate for the HMO enrollees is lower (Luft, 1981). There is some evidence that people who switch into PGPs from conventional plans have previously been lower utilizers of hospital care than those who do not switch into a PGP (Berki and Ashcraft, 1980; Eggers and Prihoda, 1982; Luft, 1981). Despite this, the average PGP enrollee is not noticeably more healthy than enrollees in conventional insurance plans (Blumberg, 1980). (This is possible because relatively recent enrollees make up only a relatively small proportion of PGP members at any point in time.) Therefore, it is unlikely that differential health status accounts for all the observed differences in hospitalization rates between enrollees in conventional plans and prepaid group practice HMOs (Luft, 1981). However, the observed differences in hospitalization rates do not necessarily reflect physicians' decisions whether to treat patients. Some of the changes in utilization rates reflect differences in the ways that treatments are provided. For instance, the design of most PGPs involves comprehensive coverage of diagnostic services in and out of the hospital, incentives to reduce hospital use, and physically convenient ambulatory facilities. Thus, for example, patient stays may be shortened by having the patient arrive the morning of the operation rather than the night before. Similarly, Kaiser-Portland reports that 35 percent of all its operative procedures were performed on a come-and-go basis, i.e., in the operating room but without a hospital admission unless complications occur (Marks et al., 1980). Such practices are becoming increasingly common in the fee-for-service sector, but the different incentives in prepaid and nonprepaid settings may explain why this cost saving technique was more quickly adopted by HMOs (Lavin, 1982). More important, things such as ambulatory diagnostic work-ups, same day (come-and-go) surgery, and come-and-stay surgery (i.e., the patient is admitted on the day of the operation) really involve minimal changes in clinical practice; they are primarily production process decisions concerning the most efficient way to carry out a specific task.

Another issue to be considered in the HMO studies is the extent to which differences may be attributable to *group practice*, rather than to the economic incentives resulting from prepayment. The relative performance of independent practice associations, which involve some financial risk sharing by independent, primarily fee-for-service prac-titioners, is much less impressive than that of PGPs (Luft, 1981). On the other hand, some fee-for-service groups seem to have hospitali-zation rates for their patients comparable to those of prepaid groups (Broida et al., 1975; Nobrega et al., 1982; Scitovksy, 1981). Why this is the case is not clear, but speculating on the cause may help clarify the different perspectives physicians and economists have on the role of incentives.

One explanation that has been offered for the low hospitalization rate in certain group practices is that the number of specialists relative to generalists is so low that the specialists are occupied with clearly necessary admissions and do not have time for the more discretionary cases. This implies that different decision criteria are used, such that the same patient would be treated differently by the specialist in such a group than by a similar specialist in solo practice. If solo practi-tioners are less busy (in general this is the case, with surgeons pre-ferring to do more procedures than they actually do), then their patients may have more extensive tests and workups, followed by hospitali-zation. By contrast, the patients in a group setting might be more likely to be told to monitor the condition over the next few months, and, if it does not improve, more aggressive treatment will be under-taken.

Notwithstanding the differences in hospitalization, patient out-comes in both styles of practice may be similar because many medical problems are self-limiting. Practitioners in both settings see their own practice styles as clinically successful. But one may ask: If both the solo and group physicians are in a fee-for-service environment, why do they not develop similar practice patterns? Put another way: What prevents the group practice from adding more specialists who, pre-sumably, would do more discretionary procedures?

We must now move back from the economist's model to something closer to clinical practice. Procedures often seen as discretionary, such as cholecystectomy, hysterectomy, and hemorrhoidectomy, are probably seen as more mundane and less challenging if only because they are so common and the patient is not in a crisis situation. If the specialists can keep busy with interesting cases by limiting the number of physicians in the group, then they probably will do so, rather than expand the group just for the sake of bigness at the cost of diluting the clinical case mix. (Note that if the group expands by adding primary physicians and thus enlarges its patient base, dilution is not an issue.) Although this scenario is plausible, one should note that the empirical base for these observations is extraordinarily thin, being limited to a handful of studies focusing on large, well-respected multispecialty group practices, often with large numbers of referral patients, such as the Mayo Clinic. Specialists in such settings may well establish rather stringent criteria for hospitalization because they have so much experience with sicker patients.

The notion of different criteria for hospitalization is very close to our original question about the impact of incentives on clinical decision making. Observational studies suffer from an inability to control for case mix, so the standard retort to the differences between HMO and fee-for-service settings is that in some subtle way HMO enrollees were healthier at the outset. Hlatky et al. (1981) undertook an important, although limited, study that controls for this problem. They sent a series of case histories of patients with various types of heart problems to a sample of board-certified cardiologists. Each physician was asked a series of questions about how he or she would manage the case and, in particular, whether certain diagnostic tests or bypass surgery would be recommended. Physicians in independent fee-for-service practice were significantly more likely than those in a prepaid group practice to recommend the tests and surgery. This finding supports the notion that clinical decision-making patterns in prepaid groups are different. Interestingly, the recommendations of the HMO physicians were similar to those of university cardiologists, making it more difficult to say that the PGP practice pattern represents inferior care. As has been noted, one cannot separate the prepayment from the group practice effects. More important, as we will soon discuss, the data do not indicate *why* or *how* the difference occurred.

Individual versus Collective Patterns of Practice

This brief review suggests that, despite the physician's general view that economic incentives do not influence clinical decisions, various bits of evidence at least are consistent with the notion that economic incentives do have an impact. The physician's perspective may be based largely on the absence of incentives in a conscious choice process. Most clinicians develop preferred ways to handle particular clinical situations and, when presented with a case, may not give much thought to alternatives or at least to the role that nonclinical factors, such as price, might have on the selection among alternatives. This section will take the issue one step further, to examine whether the influence of such incentives seems to result in clinically inappropriate choices. After all, the concerns about for-profit enterprises in medicine stem largely from the notion that care will suffer.[2] The first step in this examination is the recognition that medicine abounds with situations in which alternative clinical strategies are available with no scientific evidence indicating which is preferable. The second step is the recognition that despite this physicians may have strong preferences concerning these alternatives and that there may be a correlation between economic incentives and these preferences.

A careful review of the medical literature indicates a wide range of situations in which adequate scientific evidence does not exist to establish one treatment as definitively superior. For instance, Wennberg et al. (1980) found substantial controversies surrounding nine common surgical procedures. A great debate continues over whether certain types of coronary diseases are best managed surgically or medically (Carr et al., 1982; McIntosh, 1981). Yet in each situation individual physicians tend to prefer and to use one mode of treatment and do not behave as though there is a gray area that research evidence does not resolve.

Definitive clinical trials to narrow the gray area are extremely difficult and costly because the patient's outcome in any particular case is dependent on a host of factors in addition to the one under consideration. (Even major clinical trials often provide ambiguous results.) Thus, very large samples and sophisticated methods may be required to determine the specific gray area *situations* in which treatment A is superior to treatment B. Individual clinicians cannot undertake such studies in a systematic way. Yet many act as if the evidence were clear. I think the reason for this is threefold. First, medical training generally lacks training in research design, epide-

---

[2]Another concern is that the rise of for-profit enterprises in medicine will change the physician's perceived role so that it will no longer be that of a professional. This may entail a loss of prerogatives, status, and credibility. Furthermore, to the extent that the physician's credibility has a beneficial placebo effect on the patient, the loss of status may indirectly affect patient outcomes.

miulugy, and other analytic methods. Case reports and uncontrolled trials abound in the medical literature (McKinlay, 1981). Second, reports of new techniques are generally offered by their innovators, and the early "evaluation" is usually done by strong advocates of the technique. Although this may not lead to intentional bias in the results, various studies indicate that subsequent controlled trials often are far less supportive of the technique. (It is important to note that in most cases the technique is not found to be worse than the alternative, only not superior; i.e., it is in the gray area.) Third, although the medical literature offers little useful guidance, the practitioner constantly makes ad hoc observations that tend to support and reinforce whichever view is initially held.

Suppose the decision concerns a service that, given the available research, is truly in the gray area, such as bypass surgery for two diseased coronary arteries. For more severe disease there is clear evidence of improved survival with surgery, but the available studies are less clear for intermediate levels of obstruction. Survival rates for medical and surgical management are roughly comparable. While death rates tend to be low for both treatments, the morbidity (and costs) associated with each method differs. A physician choosing one method will tend to focus on the good outcomes, recalling that the failure rate is really no higher than for the alternative. Because patients' beliefs often are significant factors in improved outcomes (viz., the placebo effect), a physician who strongly recommends one alternative as being "superior in my experience" may well be correct because of the expectation of improvement. More important, those patients who demand a careful evaluation of the alternatives are likely to lead their physicians to react in one of two ways.[3] If they eventually follow their physician's recommendation and do less well than might be expected, their poor outcome may be blamed on insufficient trust, and the physician's preferences for not giving the patient explicit choices will be reinforced. This is often referred to as reducing cognitive dissonance. (If they do well, it merely confirms the physician's original view about the correct treatment.) However, some patients will decide against the recommended alternative and will change physicians,

[3]Some physicians encourage patients to ask questions and make choices; the increased control their patients experience may actually result in better outcomes. Careful studies of this hypothesis are not available. As has been noted earlier, this model of patient decision making reduces the physician's power, takes more time, and may be perceived as more risky. Moreover, it is probably the case that some patients want their physicians to make all the choices, although others want the reverse, and this, too, may result in self-selection (O'Donnell, 1982).

seeking out one whose views conform to their own. From the perspective of each clinician—in this case the cardiologist and the cardiac surgeon—his or her preferred treatment is better for his or her own patients. However, this is not necessarily because the treatment is truly superior but because patients select themselves among physicians.

Within the often broad gray areas concerning clinical choices, physicians may develop clear preferences for certain practice styles, preferences that have no particular scientific basis yet are self-reinforcing through a combination of placebo effects, patient selection, and the self-limiting nature of many conditions. This hypothesis provides an explanation for the wide variations in practice patterns seen among physicians, even those practicing in the same type of setting. In various studies, Wennberg and Gittelsohn have identified consistent differences over time in surgical use across small areas in New England (Wennberg and Gittelsohn, 1973, 1975, 1982). One area may have a high hysterectomy rate and a low cholecystectomy rate. The differences appear not to be related to specialty mix or population differences but to the presence of particular surgeons who use either broad or stringent indications for certain procedures. Moreover, particular surgeons are not necessarily conservative (or aggressive) across all types of procedures; instead, there seems to be little consistency. These studies also indicate that the wide variations in practice patterns tend to occur for those procedures about which the research literature provides no definitive rules, i.e., where the gray area is broad. For instance, there is little variability in the rates of herniorrhaphy, where the research is fairly definitive, in contrast to hysterectomy, where surgery often is more discretionary (Wennberg and Gittelsohn, 1982).

Wide differences in practice patterns are not limited to fee-for-service surgeons in rural New England. Studies have shown wide ranges in the use of laboratory tests, prescription drugs, X-rays, return appointments, and telephone consultations among similarly trained physicians within (not only across) such settings as university-based HMOs (Schroeder et al., 1973), large prepaid group practices (Freeborn et al., 1972), large fee-for-service multispecialty groups (Roney and Estes, 1975), and relatively small single-specialty groups (Lyle et al., 1976). Even the study by Hlatky et al. (1981), which controls for case mix by using identical case historics, shows substantial variability in the recommendations of physicians within the same types of settings. Some of the PGP cardiologists were more aggressive in their recommendations than were some independent fee-for-service practitioners. However, nearly all the cardiologists in all three types of settings recommended surgery for patients with left main artery and triple vessel disease, a recommendation clearly supported by the research literature. The variability was concentrated among the less severe cases in which the research is not definitive, further supporting the notion of differences in the gray area.

Although the wide variation in patterns within practice settings may have idiosyncratic origins, such as the teachings of an influential professor or a memorably bad experience with an alternative strategy, there also seem to be consistent patterns of care related to the method of payment and other economic incentives. The reasons for a statistical relationship between economic incentives and practice patterns are not well established. Two explanations may be offered. First, it may be that economics directly shapes the clinical patterns, so that, for example, a new physician, even one trained in a conservative, watch-and-wait style, who enters fee-for-service practice quickly recognizes that the loan will not be paid off and the yacht will be long in arriving unless he or she does more tests and procedures. (One can describe a counter example for a new partner in an HMO.) This explanation is incorporated in much of the rhetoric about fee-for-service and prepaid systems, but it rarely is reported by physicians in those settings.[4]

The second explanation focuses on the selection behavior of patients and physicians. Just as patients select a physician they think will provide the advice they desire and with whom they feel comfortable, physicians select practice patterns. By the time residency is completed, an aggressive physician probably knows an HMO is not the most conducive setting for that style of practice. In many cases choice may not be conscious. Such a physician's mentors are much more likely to be in a fee-for-service setting, and the new physician's perception is merely of following a style that clearly works. Likewise, a conservatively oriented physician may find the HMO environment more comfortable. Decisions of this type may be made primarily on the basis of collegial support; it may be difficult always to be different in one's clinical recommendations. Economic incentives probably also have a more direct influence, even if not influencing clinical decisions. Given the current structure of medical fees, a conservative practitioner in a fee-for-service environment will typically earn less than his or her

---

[4]Occasional stories of this type do appear, but they seem limited to Medicaid mills or other extreme settings. There is certainly not enough evidence of this type to explain the different practice patterns in large, mature HMOs such as Kaiser and Group Health Co-operative. The truth may be concealed because such a gross influence of economic incentives runs counter to the hallowed view of medical ethics. However, given the emotionally charged debates in this area, if this were a common problem one would have expected more evidence to have surfaced.

peers, so a switch to an HMO setting might be attractive because less use of expensive services might yield a larger year-end bonus.

The selection hypothesis also helps explain the observed positive correlation between the supply of surgeons and the incidence of surgery without resorting to a crude demand-generating model (McClure, 1982). If physicians have some implicit income target, this income level can be reached by aggressive practitioners with a small but intensively treated population base or by conservative practitioners with a larger and less intensively treated population.[5] This could result in a natural sorting process through which areas happening to have conservative practitioners are in equilibrium with low-intensity care, while areas with aggressive practitioners reach an equilibrium with high-intensity care. Of course, such a situation requires consumer insensitivity to costs (a result of extensive third-party coverage) and lack of knowledge or relative indifference to alternative treatment options. This brings us back to the question of the effectiveness of the physician as the patient's agent. However, it is important to recall that as long as we are discussing decisions in the gray area, individual physicians may firmly believe that they are following appropriate practice and that this has nothing to do with economic incentives. Furthermore, most clinicians appear to be unaware of costs or to believe that a third-party payer, not the patient, will foot the bill.

Summary and Conclusions

Much of this paper has been devoted to an attempted reconciliation of the apparently opposing opinions of physicians and economists concerning the influence of economic incentives on clinical decisions. Different approaches to empirical research and different criteria for acceptable evidence are partial explanations of the different perceptions. Perhaps more important is the central role given choice and adjustments at the margin in the economist's world view and the tendency by clinicians to view a problem as a challenge to find the one correct solution. Given such widely divergent starting points, it is difficult for economists and physicians to agree even on terminology and to discuss their differences without becoming convinced the other is totally missing the point.

On the empirical side, there is certainly evidence—concerning the

---

[5]The target-income hypothesis is hotly debated by economists who seem unable to reach a definitive conclusion on this issue yet continue to hold strong beliefs about it. Gray areas exist in medical economics as well as in medicine. See Fuchs and Newhouse (1978), Hixon (1980), Richardson (1981), Wilensky and Rossiter (1981).

adoption and use of medical technology and different practice patterns—that is consistent with the notion that economic incentives matter. Such evidence may be sufficient to convince the economist that we should examine the effects of the types of economic incentives created by different types of practices and payment settings, but it lacks the power of a randomized controlled trial to convince skeptical physicians. One of the difficulties is that from the clinician's perspective the observational studies are missing an explanation of *how* economic incentives alter practice patterns, particularly when they do not see such factors playing a role in their own experience. A possible explanation for both sets of evidence is that there is often a wide range of acceptable clinical practice, even though each clinician may believe in his or her own way. If clinicians sort themselves into different practice settings whose economic incentives are consistent with aggressive or conservative practice styles, we will observe clinical patterns that *appear* to be shaped by economics, although the clinicians themselves see no such effects.

The foregoing is a description of a relatively slow and passive process. Morever, because the medical care market has been relatively noncompetitive, there has been little active encouragement to the sorting out of physicians, let alone the evaluation of alternative clinical approaches. The gray area often is wide, but there has been relatively little exploration of how wide it might be. The situation is now beginning to change. More and more studies are being proposed or undertaken to evaluate new technologies (Bunker et al., 1982; Greenberg and Derzon, 1981; Towery and Perry, 1981). Simultaneously, the growth and development of HMOs, for-profit hospitals, health care corporations, and other organized systems provide both the means and incentive to evaluate the alternative clinical strategies in cost-effectiveness terms. This may lead to more active efforts by such organizations to use incentives or pressures to get their clinicians to alter their practice patterns. Some physicians already are beginning to view the world through the economist's eyes and to use the language of choices, trade-offs, and financial transactions (Fein, 1982). Whether such changes are desirable is a much larger question, but there can be little doubt that they are occurring.

References

Becker, Gary S. *A Treatise on the Family.* Cambridge: Harvard University Press, 1981.

Berki, S. E., and Ashcraft, Marie L. F. "HMO Enrollment: Who Joins and Why: A Review of the Literature." *Milbank Memorial Fund Quarterly/Health and Society* 58:4 (Fall 1980):558-632.

Blumberg, Mark S. "Health Status and Health Care Use by Type of Private Health Coverage." *Milbank Memorial Fund Quarterly/Health and Society* 58:4 (Fall 1980):633-55.

Blumberg, Mark S. "Provider Price Charges for Improved Health Care Use." In *Health Handbook.* Edited by George K. Chako. Amsterdam: North-Holland, 1979.

Broida, Joel et al. "Impact of Membership in an Enrolled Prepaid Population on Utilization of Health Services in a Group Practice." *The New England Journal of Medicine* 292:15 (10 April 1975):780-83.

Bunker, John P. "A Comparison of Operations and Surgeons in the United States and in England and Wales. *The New England Journal of Medicine* 282:3 (15 January 1970):135-44.

Bunker, John P., Jinnet Fowles, and Ralph Schffarzick. "Evaluation of Medical Technology Strategies." *The New England Journal of Medicine* 306:10-11 (11, 18 March 1982):620-624, 687-92.

California Medical Association. *1974 Revision of the 1969 California Relative Value Studies.* San Francisco: Sutter Publications, 1975.

Caper, Philip. "Competition and Health Care: A New Trojan Horse?" *The New England Journal of Medicine* 306:15 (15 April 1982):928-29.

Carr, Kenneth W., Robert L. Engler, and John Ross, Jr. "Do Coronary Artery Bypass Operations Prolong Life?" *Western Journal of Medicine* 136:4 (April 1982):295-308.

Childs, Alfred W., and Hunter, E. Diane. "Non-Medical Factors Influencing the Use of Diagnostic X-ray by Physicians." *Medical Care* 10:4 (July/August 1972):323-35.

Cook, Wallace H. "Profile of the Permanente Physician." In *The Kaiser-Permanente Medical Care Program: A Symposium.* Edited by Anne R. Somers. New York: Commonwealth Fund, 1971.

Eddy, David M. "Clinical Policies and the Quality of Clinical Practice." *The New England Journal of Medicine* 307:6 (5 August 1982):343-47.

Eggers, Paul W., and Prihoda, Ronald. "Pre-Enrollment Reimbursement Patterns of Medicare Beneficiaries Enrolled in 'At Risk' HMOs." *Health Care Financing Review* 4:1 (September 1982):55-74.

Fein, Rashi. "What is Wrong with the Language of Medicine." *The New England Journal of Medicine* 306:14 (8 April 1982):863-64.

Feldstein, Martin S. "Econometric Studies of Health Economics." In *Frontiers of Quantitative Economics.* Edited by M. Intriligator and D. Kendrick. Amsterdam: North-Holland, 1974.

Fineberg, Harvey V. "Clinical Chemistries: The High Cost of Low-Cost Diagnostic Tests." In *Medical Technology: The Culprit Behind Health Care Costs?* Proceedings of the 1977 Sun Valley Forum on National Health. National Center for Health Services Research, DHEW Publ. No. (PHS) 79-3216, Washington, D.C., 1979.

Freeborn, Donald K. et al. "Determinants of Medical Care Utilization: Physician's Use of Laboratory Services." *American Journal of Public Health* 62:6 (June 1972):846-53.

Fuchs, Victor R., and Newhouse, Joseph P. "The Conference and Unresolved Problems." *Journal of Human Resources* 13 Suppl. (1978):5-20.

Greenberg, Barbara, and Derzon, Robert A. "Determining Health Insurance Coverage of Technology: Problems and Options." *Medical Care* 19:10 (October 1981):967-78.

Griner, Paul F. et al. "Selection and Interpretation of Diagnostic Tests and Procedures." *Annals of Internal Medicine* 94:5 (Part 2), (May 1981):553-600.

Grossman, Michael. *The Demand for Health: A Theoretical and Empirical Investigation.* New York: Columbia University Press for the National Bureau of Economic Research, 1972.

Grossman, Michael. "The Demand for Health After a Decade." *Journal of Health Economics* 1:1 (1982):1-3.

Hixon, Jesse S., ed. *The Target Income Hypothesis*. Bureau of Health Manpower, DHEW Publ. No. (HRS) 80-27. Washington, D.C.: U.S. Government Printing Office, 1980.

Hlatky, Mark A., E. Botvinick, and B. Brundage. "A Controlled Comparison of Cardiac Diagnostic Test Use in a Health Maintenance Organization." Presented at the Annual Meeting of the Robert Wood Johnson Clinical Scholars. San Antonio, Tex., 11-14 November 1981.

Lavin, John H. "Same-Day Surgery: Why Everyone Is Learning to Love It." *Medical Economics* 59:12 (7 June 1982):110 ff.

Lewin, Lawrence S., Robert A. Derzon, and Rhea Margulies. "Investor-Owned and Nonprofits Differ in Economic Performance." *Hospitals* 55 (1 July 1981):52-58.

Luft, Harold S. *Health Maintenance Organizations: Dimensions of Performance*. New York: Wiley-Interscience, 1981.

Lyle, Carl B. et al. "Practice Habits in a Group of Eight Internists." *Annals of Internal Medicine* 84:5 (May 1976):594-601.

Marks, Sylvia D. et al. "Ambulatory Surgery in an HMO: A Study of Costs, Quality of Care and Satisfaction." *Medical Care* 18:2 (February 1980):127-46.

Martin, Albert R. "Common and Correctable Errors in Diagnostic Test Ordering." *Western Journal of Medicine* 136:5 (May 1982):456-61.

McClure, Walter. "Toward Development and Application of a Qualitative Theory of Hospital Utilization." *Inquiry* 19:2 (Summer 1982):117-35.

McIntosh, H. D. *Overview of Aortocoronary Bypass Grafting for the Treatment of Coronary Artery Disease: An Internist's Perspective*. Washington, D.C.: National Center for Health Care Technology, 1981.

McKinlay, John B. "From 'Promising Report' to 'Standard Procedure': Seven Stages in the Career of a Medical Innovation." *Milbank Memorial Fund Quarterly/Health and Society* 59:3 (Summer 1981):374-411.

McNeil, Barbara J. et al. "On the Elicitation of Preferences for Alternative Therapies." *The New England Journal of Medicine* 306:21 (27 May 1982):1259-62.

McNeil, Barbara J., and Adelstein, S. James. "The Values of Case Finding in Hypertensive Renovascular Disease." *The New England Journal of Medicine* 293:5 (31 July 1975):221-26.

Moloney, Thomas W., and Rogers, David E. "Medical Technology—A Different View of the Contentious Debate Over Costs." *The New England Journal of Medicine* 301:26 (27 December 1979):1413-19.

Nobrega, Fred T. et al. "Hospital Use in a Fee-for-Service System." *Journal of the American Medical Association* 247:6 (12 February 1982):806-10.

O'Donnell, Walter E. "Let's Stop Ducking Decisions on Patient Care." *Medical Economics* 59:14 (5 July 1982):32ff.

Pauker, Stephen G., and Kassirer, Jerome P. "Therapeutic Decision Making: A Cost-Benefit Analysis." *The New England Journal of Medicine* 293:5 (31 July 1975):229-34.

Pauly, Mark V. *Doctors and Their Workshops: Economic Models of Physician Behavior*. Chicago: University of Chicago Press, 1980.

Relman, Arnold S. "The New Medical-Industrial Complex." *The New England Journal of Medicine* 303:17 (23 October 1980):963-70.

Richardson, J. "The Inducement Hypothesis: That Doctors Generate Demand for Their Own Services." In *Health, Economics and Health Economics*. Edited by Jacques Van der Gaag and Mark Perlman. Amsterdam: North-Holland, 1981.

Roney, James G., and Estes, Hilliard D. "Automated Health Testing in a Medical Group Practice." *Public Health Reports* 90:2 (March/April 1975):126-32.

Saward, Ernest, and Sorensen, Andrew. "Competition, Profit and the HMO." *The New England Journal of Medicine* 306:15 (15 April 1982):929-31.

Schroeder, Steven A., and Showstack, Jonathan A. "Financial Incentives to Perform Medical Procedures and Laboratory Tests: Illustrative Models of Office Practice." *Medical Care* 16:4 (April 1978):289-98.

Schroeder, Steven A. et al. "Use of Laboratory Tests and Pharmaceuticals: Variation Among Physicians and Effects of Cost Audit on Subsequent Use." *Journal of the American Medical Association* 225:8 (20 August 1973):969-73.

Scitovsky, Anne A. "The Use of Medical Services Under Prepaid and Fee-for-Service Group Practice." Social Science and Medicine 15C (1981):107-16.

Showstack, Jonathan A., and Schroeder, Steven A. "The Cost-Effectiveness of Upper Gastrointestinal Endoscopy." Background Paper No. 2, Case Studies of Medical Technologies—Case Study 8: Implications of Cost-Effectiveness Analysis of Medical Technology. Washington, D.C.: Office of Technology Assessment, U.S. Congress, May 1981.

Showstack, Jonathan A. et al. "Fee-for-Service Physician Payment: Analysis of Current Methods and Their Development." *Inquiry* 16:3 (Fall 1979):230-46.

Towery, O. B., and Perry, Seymour. "The Scientific Basis for Coverage Decisions by Third-Party Payers." *Journal of the American Medical Association* 245:1 (2 January 1981):59-61.

Wennberg, John E., John P. Bunker, and Benjamin Barnes. "The Need for Assessing the Outcome of Common Clinical Practices." *Annual Review of Public Health* 1 (1980):277-95.

Wennberg, John E., and Gittelsohn, Alan. "Health Care Delivery in Maine I: Patterns of Use of Common Surgical Procedures." *Journal of Maine Medical Association* 66:5 (May 1975):123-30, 49.

Wennberg, John E., and Gittelsohn, Alan. "Small Variations in Health Care Delivery." *Science* 182:4117 (14 December 1973):1102-8.

Wennberg, John E., and Gittelsohn, Alan. "Variations in Medical Care Among Small Areas." *Scientific American* 246:4 (April 1982):120ff.

Wilensky, Gail Roggin, and Rossiter, Louis F. "The Magnitude and Determinants of Physician-Initiated Visits in the United States. In *Health, Economics and Health Economics*. Edited by Jacques van der Gaag and Mark Perlman. Amsterdam: North-Holland, 1981.

Wilson, Edward O. "The Ergonomics of Caste in the Social Insects." *American Economic Review* 68:6 (December 1978):25-36.

Ethical Dilemmas of For-Profit Enterprise in Health Care

Robert M. Veatch

The practice of medicine should not be commercialized nor treated as a commodity of trade.

—AMA *Judicial Council Opinions and Reports*, 1969

The type of financial arrangement between a physician and a hospital, corporation or other lay body is important and relevant in determining whether or not such an arrangement is ethical. We further believe that the amount of a physician's income or whether or not an institution is making a profit on his services is irrelevent in whether an arrangement is ethical.

—AMA Board of Trustees, 1957

The rapid evolution of for-profit corporate delivery of health care over the past few years poses critical questions for those interested in the ethics of health care delivery. The development of commercial dialysis centers, corporate for-profit hospital chains, and other health care delivery systems linking health care to profit-making enterprise raises critical sociological, legal, economic, administrative, and political issues. In addition to all of these it challenges some of the most fundamental ethical presuppositions of both the business and the health care communities.

The relationship between business and professional health care has always been an ambivalent one. Organized medicine in the United States has never condemned outright the practice of medicine within a profit-making context. Yet over the years, beginning with concern about restraining unorthodox practitioners and continuing in debates over physician control of pharmacies, patents, advertising, and financial arrangements in group practice, organized medicine has constantly been nervous about the pestilential taint of commercialization.

History of the Ethics Controversy

The International Context

If we are to understand the new ethical problems that may emerge with the evolution of for-profit enterprise in health care, it is worth, first, examining the history of the ethical controversy over some historical analogues of that relationship and then attempting to synthesize a description of the potential problems to be anticipated. That history reveals that ambiguity has long troubled those trying to understand the relation of medicine to for-profit commercial enterprise.

Confucian medicine in ancient China was essentially an art practiced within a family. Each family had someone skilled in medicine who could look after his kin, acting out of the traditional virtues of compassion, applied humaneness, and filial piety. The later professionalization of medicine, so that financial transactions necessarily became a part of the practice of the art, was widely viewed as the beginning of the downfall of the lofty ideals of medicine.[1]

The medical literature of ancient Greece is filled with examples of instances in which it is implied that the motivation of the practitioner might have been something less than applied humaneness. A search of the Hippocratic corpus to find evidence that a philanthropic attitude is essential in medicine proves fruitless.[2] Galen bemoans the fact that philanthropy is the inspiration for only a minority of physicians, because the majority pursue money, honor, or glory.[3] It was standard advice for physicians to choose carefully whom they would accept as patients lest they take on a hopeless case and have their reputations tarnished and their market potential jeopardized by their failure.

By the time of the beginnings of modern Anglo-American medical ethics, we still find little attention being paid to the ethics of the business and commercial dimensions of professional health care. One searches the long, detailed Code of Thomas Percival of 1797 in vain for relevant material. This is true even though this code, which was to become the foundation of both British and American medical ethics, was originally written in response to an unsavory feud among physicians, surgeons, and apothecaries at the Manchester Infirmary in England, a fight having the tone of a cutthroat, corporate boardroom machination.[4] It was not until the twentieth century that the professional documents of Anglo-American medical ethics began dealing with the specifics of the ethical conundrum of the possibility that medical practice might, to the uninitiated, look something like a business.

A recent British Medical Association document opens its discussion of the topic by stating: "A general ethical principle is that a doctor should not associate himself with commerce in such a way as to let it influence; or appear to influence, his attitude towards the treatment of his patients."[5] This is followed by specific prohibitions and approvals. For example, physicians are to avoid having a financial interest in the sale of pharmaceuticals or writing testimonials. The concern not only focuses on the risk that commercial involvement could affect decisions but also extends to concern about the appearance of being influenced.

The Australian Medical Association Code of Ethics has the same principle stated verbatim, with similar examples, followed by an impossibly convoluted set of sentences attempting to walk a tightrope on the subject of ownership of pharmaceutical companies.[6]

The American Medical Association

The codes of the American Medical Association (AMA) have shown similar ambivalence through the years. To be sure, the positions adopted by the AMA do not always reflect the current views of the American public or even those of American physicians. They surely do not describe actual behavior in all cases. They are, however, the most important consensus statements of organized professional medicine in the United States. As such, they do normally reflect the ideal of what most physicians, at least those who participate in AMA activities, consider to be ethical conduct for physicians.

The early codes of the AMA, beginning with the original versions passed at the convention in Philadelphia in 1847, state flat prohibitions of certain behavior that everyone seemed to think obviously made the physician too much like a businessman and therefore in danger of ethical misconduct. These codes concentrated on prohibiting advertising, holding of patents, and dispensing "secret nostrums." Acting like a businessman was considered unacceptable, but even appearing like one seemed to be as much a cause of concern. During this period medical practitioners whom we now would identify as practic-

ing orthodox medicine were very concerned about separating themselves from quacks and charlatans, who often engaged in commercial
tactics.

Advertising   The AMA in 1847 stated that: "It is derogatory to the
dignity of the profession, to resort to public advertisements or private
cards or handbills, inviting the attention of individuals affected with
particular diseases. . . ."[7] The same declaration is repeated verbatim
in the revision of 1903 and in new, even stronger language in the
1912 revision.[8] The objection was clearly to the businesslike style of
advertising, regardless of content. Publicizing successes, inviting laymen to witness operations, and boasting of cures were deemed "the
ordinary practices of empirics [quacks], and are highly reprehensible
in a regular physician."

By 1957, with a much shortened set of principles, the prohibition
had been reduced to the mandate that the physician "should not solicit
patients."[9] The interpretation began to get more subtle. Spurred by
the Federal Trade Commission's (FTC) suit claiming that prohibition
on solicitation was restraining free trade, the AMA began emphasizing that what it wanted to prohibit was "deceptive practices," "false
or misleading statements," and the "creation of unjustified expectations." In short, the AMA's position had shifted to one that any good
Madison Avenue advertising executive might endorse. What began
as an effort to distinguish medical professionals from quacks, and
others whom they tried to identify with mere business people, ended
up making them demand to be recognized (by the FTC and others) as
free-market competitors at their best.

Patents   A similar progression is seen with the AMA's statements
on physician holding of patents. The original position in 1847 was
blunt: "It is derogatory to professional character . . . for a physician
to hold a patent for any surgical instrument or medicine. . . ."[10] By
1971 the practice was acceptable, but nervousness was apparent in
the qualifications and warnings.[11] With the major revision in 1981
all signs of ethical doubt about patents had disappeared. It is now
stated bluntly that: "It is not unethical for a physician to patent a
surgical or diagnostic instrument."[12]

Dispensing Pharmaceuticals and Receiving Rebates   The older codes
explicitly condemn not only the holding of patents but also the prescribing of "secret nostrums." Originally the concern was over the
secrecy as such, a point that will be important later when we contrast

professional medical ethics with business ethics.[13] It was more important to distinguish the physician from a charlatan than from a businessman. That same condemnation appeared in the AMA documents into the 1970s when it finally disappeared.

Far more important and difficult is the question of whether physicians could sell more orthodox pharmaceuticals. It has long been recognized that physicians who sell their own remedies have a potential conflict of interest. The codes seem to express two concerns: that financial pressures might influence prescribing and that there should be a proper division of labor with pharmacists. From the time of the 1957 revision it was accepted that: "Drugs, remedies or appliances may be dispensed or supplied by the physician provided it is in the best interests of the patient."[14] Because of the potential appearance of conflict of interest and also probably to avoid tensions with pharmacists, the AMA urged physicians "to avoid the regular dispensing and the retail sale of drugs to patients whenever the drug needs of patients can be met adequately by local ethical pharmacies."[15] For similar reasons accepting rebates on prescriptions and appliances has been consistently condemned as unethical.[16]

In 1947 the ophthalmologists aggravated the AMA Judicial Council by presenting so many schemes for rebates that the Council was uncharacteristically exasperated in its response.[17] Among the tasks of the Council was review of ethical queries from members. Ophthalmologists were seeking ways in which they could receive some remuneration, beyond their usual professional fee, for prescribing eye glasses. Rebates from opticians were a common practice. The Council's response was curt: "By far the largest number of requests for information on approval were received from ophthalmologists who have submitted practically every conceivable plan to circumvent the section of the Principles of Medical Ethics concerning rebates. . . . It is strange that year after year more communications regarding these practices come from members of this particular field than from any other. . . . No matter how prevalent these practices may have become, they are still unethical."

Fee Splitting   Closely related to dispensing of pharmaceuticals and receiving rebates is the problem of fee splitting. It has been fundamental to professional medical ethics since 1912 that fee splitting is unethical, "detrimental to the public good and degrading to the profession," according to the 1912 code. Originally the emphasis was on secrecy in the splitting of fees, but since the 1950s the practice itself, secret or not, has been condemned. It is viewed as an unacceptable induoomont that "violates the patient's trust that the physician will not exploit his dependence upon him. . . ."[18]

Recently, the economist Mark Pauly has argued forcefully that the *absence* of fee splitting might also produce undue inducements—in this case inducements for the generalist to treat patients who ought to be referred.[19] He concludes that fee splitting ought to be viewed as ethical. While such a conclusion is debatable, at least it suggests that the unanimous, vitriolic condemnation of fee splitting may have latent functions, perhaps, such as maintenance of the idea that the health care professional is significantly different from a business person, for whom commissions, royalties, finder's fees, and the like are standard.

Ownership of Health Facilities and Corporate Relations   The problems examined thus far—advertising, patents, rebates, and fee splitting—constitute the classic issues of the ethics of physician finances. The answers, at least for a time, were simple: Behaving like a rational, self-interested businessman was unethical. Gradually, as the complexities of the business of practicing medicine became more clear, qualifications began to cloud the picture. These matters are still relatively simple in comparison with the ethical problems of corporate for-profit delivery of health care, in which the ambivalence of the physician/business relation is seen full blown. It is in this context that the ethical tensions of practicing medicine in a for-profit corporate context begin to have their closest analogues with more traditional issues in medical ethics.

The first major set of ethical issues is physician ownership of health care facilities. It is now clear that the AMA has concluded that it is acceptable for physicians to own pharmacies[20]; hospitals[21]; nursing homes[22]; and, by implication, laboratories.[23] It also is clear, however, that in all these cases the AMA considers it unethical for a physician to be influenced in his or her medical practice by such ownership. Until the redrafting of the AMA code of ethics in 1980, there was a strict prohibition on any arrangement whereby physicians would profit on investments in proportion to the amount of work they referred to the laboratory.[24] Thus, physicians could in fact profit from the referrals to pharmacies, nursing homes, hospitals, and laboratories that they owned but were held to a standard in which they acted as if they would not, and in no case could they receive a fee or return on investment directly linked to the business they generated. Still it was considered acceptable for them to share in the profits of the facilities they owned, including the profits they knew they were generating from their own medical practices.

The links between the practice of medicine and the corporate commercial interest in health care delivery are not always as simple as straightforward ownership by a physician. With physician ownership, professional associations such as the AMA could at least appeal to the recognition that physicians had control of the corporations with which they had financial ties. More complex corporate relations with for-profit enterprise may involve physicians in positions where they exercise much less direct control.

The versions of the *Judicial Council Opinions and Reports* of the late 1960s and early 1970s place great emphasis on the ethical problems of physicians practicing within the context of lay-owned corporations or where lay groups profited directly from their service.[25]

The privilege of healing the sick as a profession is a right granted only to those properly qualified and licensed by the state. It is a privilege belonging only to the medical profession. It is a sacrifice of professional dignity that this exclusive right of medicine is so often sold for individual gain or its possessor deprived of it against his will. In increasing numbers, physicians are disposing of their professional attainments to lay organizations under terms which permit a direct profit from the fees or salaries paid for their services to accrue to the lay bodies employing them. Such a procedure is absolutely destructive of that personal responsibility and relationship which is essential to the best interest of the patient.[26]

The Judicial Council gives three examples. The first is hardly clear-cut: salaries or fees paid to the physician by insurance companies in workman's compensation cases in which the fees allegedly are below the legal fees on which a premium is based. The other two, however, are more directly relevant to for-profit health care enterprise: hospitals collecting fees for professional services of staff physicians and absorbing them as hospital income, and universities employing full-time hospital staffs and sharing such fees for the professional care of patients "as to net the university no small profit."

Several things are worth noting. First, the Judicial Council is concerned that the right and the dignity of the profession is assaulted by such practices of lay corporations. Second, it believes that such lay involvement destroys professional responsibility and is contrary to the best interest of patients. Finally, underlying much of the Council's concern is a commitment to the maintenance of professional control. The Council's conclusion, one apparently relevant to for-profit health care enterprises, is that: "A physician should not dispose of his professional attainments or services to any hospital, corporation or lay body by whatever name called or however organized under terms or conditions which permit the sale of the services of that physician by such an agency for a fee."[27]

The recent evolution of for-profit enterprise in health care has the potential of engaging the physician in a number of capacities: as an employee of a for-profit hospital or other corporation, as an independent practitioner referring patients to the for-profit corporation for certain medical services, and as an owner of the for-profit corporation. The concern about the dignity of the profession might be a particular problem where physicians are owners. The other forms of participation, however, seem to present even greater difficulty because physicians could lose control over medical practices, abandoning responsibility to lay people.

By the late 1970s all of this AMA language pertaining to physician relations with lay-owned corporations disappeared, and it was entirely absent from the major revision of the document in 1981. As far as this author has been able to determine, there was no formal change of policy or reversal by any official AMA body. Rather, the warnings against involvement with lay-dominated corporations simply were omitted, leaving the concerned reader to speculate whether the AMA had accommodated the relationship or simply thought it not worth attention any longer.

A Summary of the Professional Physician Stance

This brief history makes it clear that the attitude of American professional organized medicine toward the commercial aspects of health care has been a complex and ambivalent one. From this complex and shifting pattern of professional attitudes it may be possible to glean a pattern or at least a set of principles that informs the Judicial Council and other AMA pronouncements.

Basic Principles of the Professional Stance

Service to the Patient   Historically, all of medical ethics in the Hippocratic tradition, including that of Anglo-American medical ethics, affirms as the basic principle the idea that the physician should use his or her judgment to do what he or she thinks will benefit the patient. It is not surprising, therefore, that the professional stance on the finances of medical practice is normally legitimated by appeal to the welfare of the patient. The condemnation of physicians who allow lay corporations to profit directly from their services is thus characteristic when it ends by arguing that prohibiting such an arrangement is "essential to the best interests of the patient." The AMA's brief in its defense against the FTC's charge that it unlawfully restrained physician advertising was argued in similar terms.

Physicians' financial interests are often consistent with many of the practices labeled by the AMA as ethically required. Control of advertising and prohibition of lay profits from professional services are obvious examples. This had led some to suggest that self-interested motives have led organized medicine to label certain business practices unethical. In fact the author of an anthropological study of Chinese medical ethics argues that the primary function of medical ethics is the control of financial and other rewards of professional service.[28] Pauly's analysis of fee splitting, in contrast to the professional physician literature, simply assumes that physicians will primarily pursue self-interest and only at the margin be influenced by patient welfare.

Holders of these contrasting attitudes about the role of commitment to patient welfare and self-interest fail to grasp what sociologists sometimes refer to as the relationship between the latent and manifest functions of positions adopted and behavior undertaken. There is good reason to believe professionals when they say they are committed to the welfare of their patients. However, this does not necessarily mean that the positions they take about what serves the welfare of their patients may not be influenced by other, more hidden, even subconscious agendas and value frameworks unique to their professional group. It also does not exclude the possibility that what they legitimately believe will serve patient welfare may also serve other interests as well, including their own.

Recently there has been an increasing recognition that the ethics of physician practice is more complex than simply serving the interests of patients. Rights language is increasingly replacing welfare language. The ethical responsibilities of physicians are increasingly being defined in terms of the rights of patients, instead of in terms of the welfare of patients. The rights language appears formally for the first time in the AMA principles in the revision of 1980. The rights of colleagues and other health care professionals are explicitly affirmed as well as those of patients. It is in the same spirit that the 1981 *Opinions of the Judicial Council* with regard to patents affirms the "sound doctrine that one is entitled to protect his discovery." Thus, perhaps, part of the softening of the professional opposition to the business imagery is related to the increasing recognition of the legitimacy of self-interest of health care professionals.

Physician Control of Decision Making and Fees   Within the context of the dominating principle of service to the patient and often legitimated by it, a second important theme running through the AMA literature is the importance of professional control of decision making and of fees. In no case is the physician's involvement with business condemned when the professional is able to maintain such control. However, paragraphs dealing with professional involvement repeatedly include the warning that professionals must not lose control of their sphere of responsibility.

To the extent that this is a principle underlying the response of professional physician organizations to for-profit health care, it seems clear that physicians will be particularly uncomfortable when the relation is one of the physician as employee of a lay-owned corporation. There may well be less concern when physicians themselves are owners of such enterprises.

Acceptance of Profit Motive   A third basic theme one can deduce from the AMA literature is not stated as boldly but represents an inescapable conclusion. Nowhere in all of the professional literature of Anglo-American medical ethics is there any condemnation of the profit motive in the practice of medicine. While ancient Confucian medicine could look down on those who practiced medicine for financial reward, American medicine is much more open to profit. In fact, as was seen in the second epigraph of this paper, the AMA has viewed the question of whether an institution is making a profit on the physician's services as irrelevant to whether the arrangement is ethical.

Suspicion of Commercialization   Despite this openness to the profit motive, American professional organized medicine has shown a strong and stubborn resistance to anything it takes to imply the commercialization of medical practice. As recently as 1981 the AMA Judicial Council condemned commercialization (while affirming the right to make a "fair compensation").[29]

An Interpretation of the Professional Stance

The question of immediate importance for this essay is the relevance of this professional history and the principles derived from it for the evolution of for-profit enterprise in health care delivery. While some of the elements have clear connections with the recent development of commercial hemodialysis and hospital chains owned by large profit-making corporations, there is a sense of discontinuity—that something of moral significance is at stake beyond the ethical problems faced by the small-town general practitioner whose income was tied to his or her medical advice. Two major elements seem to be important in the recent developments: commercial motivation of for-profit enterprise and the subordination of medicine to the objectives of lay people. As we have seen, neither of these by itself is a new concern for physician ethics. Each has arisen at many points in the history of modern medicine, but neither has presented insurmountable obstacles to the business of practicing medicine.

We have seen that commercialization is uniformly frowned upon, but profit-making has been tolerated and even accepted as an appropriate part of medical practice. Thus, a physician practicing medicine in a profit-making context has never been viewed as unacceptable. In those cases, however, the emphasis has always been on the maintenance of professional autonomy within the sphere of medical decision making.

On the other hand, it is clear that medicine has from time to time been subordinated to the objectives of lay people—in missionary medicine, military medicine, and similar settings. The church has routinely incorporated medical practice into its mission efforts, sometimes with a rather explicit understanding that health care is a recruitment technique used to involve potential converts in much larger objectives. Likewise, the military has sometimes expected physicians to practice traditional medicine appropriate to the needs of patients but also at times to serve propaganda and other strategic objectives. The case of Howard Levy, a dermatologist recruited for the Green Berets to use his skill to train people to win support of Viet Nam villagers, is an example.[30] In both of these situations physicians could practice medicine pursuing the traditional objectives of the profession with little or no compromise. Possibly that helps explain the relative lack of controversy. Of course, protests from the profession did begin to emerge. The major difference between these lay uses of medicine and the corporate practice of medicine, however, may well be their not-for-profit, charitable, or public service nature.

It may be that, although both profit-making commercialization of medicine and subordination to lay objectives have taken place in the past and have raised concern on the part of physicians, each element taken alone was tolerable and could be accommodated within professional ethics. The new dimension of the for-profit commercial corporations may be the convergence of these two features, each of which traditionally has been troublesome for physicians in the view of organized medicine. Never before have they had to face in a major way the commercialization of medicine and the subordination of medicine to lay objectives in the same enterprise. Lay administrators, some of whom have been trained in business management, have not provided a similar conflict because the overall mission of the traditional hospital was a not-for-profit one or a charitable one, and, in any case, as the sociology of medicine makes clear, a dual line of authority has traditionally been maintained, so that physicians have retained decision-making authority over areas related to patient care and medical practice.

Corporate medicine as practiced by company physicians is the closest analogue and that is a small-scale development in comparison with the potential of for-profit enterprise. Traditional organized medicine, if this is correct, was capable of tentative accommodation to the complex realities of the business of medicine when some commercialization was involved, provided physicians retained dominance in medical decision making. It was also willing to accommodate the realities of lay control (i.e., trustees, administrators, and the sponsoring organization's mission), provided the objectives were civic or charitable. The two elements coming together, however, may well pose new challenges that will test to its utmost the ability of the profession to accommodate. This may partially explain why the for-profit hospital typically increases physician membership on hospital boards.

Physicians Compared with Other Professionals

The problems faced by physicians who practice medicine in the setting of a for-profit enterprise are likely to be similar to those faced by other professionals. A full examination of the histories of the ethics of other professional groups has not been possible, but the results of a limited exploration have not been encouraging. The professional groups of accountants, engineers, lawyers, and public policy analysts have been examined to determine if their longer history of dealings with large profit-making corporations could shed light on potential moral tensions between the professional and his or her employers. It became apparent quickly that serious disanalogies among the professions limit the usefulness of the comparison. Certified public accountants (CPAs), for example, have in their dominant code (the "Rules of Conduct" of the American Institute of Certified Public Accountants) strong statements requiring the independence of accountants.[31] No financial ties of any kind are permitted with the enterprise for whom the accountant is expressing an opinion on financial statements. There is no direct condemnation of a CPA serving as an employee of a corporation, but such a relationship clearly would be counterproductive to certain functions of CPAs. The primary purpose of the CPA is to assure outsiders of the reliability of financial statements of a corporation. Financial independence is essential for the certification to be trustworthy. It is thus in the nature of the role relation that the accountant be independent. No similar role requirements force a physician to be independent of an enterprise providing health care.

Engineers, by contrast, have long since accommodated to performing their work as employees of for-profit corporations. Several different societies of engineers serve as professional organizations for various speciality branches of engineering. Several have no formal codes at all. Six groups (including those for chemical, industrial, agricultural, civil, mechanical, and ceramic engineers) subscribe to the "Canons of Ethics of Engineers" of the Engineers' Council for Professional Development, the umbrella organization of the professional societies of engineers. None of their codes, including the "Canons" of the Engineers' Council, raises any question about an engineer working as an employee of a corporation. In fact, an employer-employee relationship is assumed. The sections dealing with the engineer's relation with the public and with employers provide the closest analogies that have been located to the kinds of problems a physician might face if employed by a for-profit corporation owning a hospital or other health care facility. These sections make clear that the engineer has a direct obligation to the public to have a proper regard for safety, health, and welfare; to extend public knowledge; and to "indicate to his employer or client the adverse consequences to be expected if his engineering judgment is overruled."[32] The essence of the engineering position is clear; employment in a for-profit corporation may pose ethical problems calling forth the ethical integrity of the engineer, but with diligence any such problems can be overcome.

Since some engineers own their own engineering corporations, we might hope to find here some guidance on cases where physicians might become owners of for-profit health care facilities. Such a hope would be frustrated, however. Other than these vague comments on the engineer's obligation to the public, there are no comments on potential conflict between the engineer-owner's commercial self-interest and the interest of the client.

Lawyers represent an intermediate case. There is some literature on the practice of law in a corporate setting.[33] It reveals that lawyers have a long history of employment within the corporate nexus, yet emphasizes their independence. The older version of the Canons of Professional Ethics of the American Bar Association includes a relevant provision originally adopted in 1928. This provision states that "the professional services of a lawyer should not be controlled or exploited by any lay agency, personal or corporate, which intervene between the client and the lawyer."[34] The same provision makes clear that it is acceptable for a lawyer to be employed by an organization but then goes on to place a critical limitation prohibiting legal services to persons within the organization. An important feature of providing health care by corporate for-profit enterprises is that the recipient of the professional's services is an individual—not the corporation itself. In fact the corporation may have a financial interest in seeing that the individual client gets something other than the best medical services. By contrast most professionals—engineers, accountants, and corporate lawyers—are providing their professional services directly for the benefit of the corporation. If they have a responsibility to outsiders, it is to some vague "public," not generally to individual consumers of their services.

Lawyers, like physicians, might theoretically provide their services to individuals, say members of an organization, while on the payroll of that organization. It is this that the AMA Canons of Professional Ethics (in effect until 1976) expressly prohibits.[35] Thus, examples of situations directly analogous to the problems of providing health care in a corporate setting did not arise in the lawyer's context, at least until recently. A search of early ethical opinions from the Committee on Ethics and Professional Responsibility of the AMA failed to reveal any cases of relevance.[36]

It appears that many of the more critical problems anticipated in the health care sphere either do not arise in accounting, engineering, and law or are not considered insurmountable. Problems of constraining services deemed by the professional to be necessary but rejected by the corporation as inefficient do not get addressed, for example. Neither do problems of excluding clients who cannot pay market prices for the professional's services. In none of the other professions do the problems of professionals functioning as owners of a profit-making enterprise get attention, either because they do not play that role or because the problems arising when they do play it are apparently not considered serious. It appears that little will be gained by examining further the codes of other professional groups. Their situations are too different. They have not addressed adequately the problems when they are analogous, and the services at stake are arguably morally different. Even if engineering or accounting services are justifiably distributed by the use of market mechanisms, it is not clear that health care services would be.

A Philosophical Evaluation of the Problem

Problems with Evaluations Based on Professional Codes

The commission for this paper emphasized examination of the ways in which physician involvement in for-profit health care enterprise has been addressed in professional codes of ethics. We have seen that there is a great deal of concern, much marginally relevant material from an earlier era, and a great deal of residual ambivalence of the professional codes to any long-term resolution of the problems of concern to the Institute of Medicine.

In the first place, it is clear that the codes have shifted considerably over the years from an explicit antipathy to the business connotations of such matters as advertising to the adoption of a position that seems little different from that of any ethically practiced business concern. More critically, it is not clear how the particular positions of professional groups should be taken into account by the broader public in formulating policy, even when those positions are stated unambiguously.

At most, the positions expressed in professional codes reflect the moral consensus of the profession. More realistically they reflect the consensus of the segment of the profession that actively participates in organized professional matters. It is well known that such activists do not necessarily reflect the full range of the members of the profession. Even if they did, however, there is a broader philosophical problem in relying on the codes articulated by professional groups for determining the proper norms for ethical relationships between professionals and the broader public.

In spite of the arguments that abound about the latent, more self-serving functions of professional codes, this author is convinced that it is reasonable to take these codes as good-faith expressions of what professions consider to be ethical conduct for members of their groups. The fact that the codes reflect a good-faith consensus of what the professional groups take to be ethical conduct is not enough to legitimate the use of the codes for resolving matters of professional ethics. For a rule of ethical conduct to be justified it must conform to a set of basic ethical principles derived from sources that are far more universal and far more fundamental than mere professional consensus. Exactly what those sources are remains a matter of dispute. The great religious traditions see the basic principles as coming from God, perhaps reflected in moral natural laws. Our founding fathers saw them as self-evident truths. Some philosophers see them as derived from a basic social contract. In any case these basic principles are something shared by an entire moral community; they are not the exclusive property of a group, professional or otherwise, within the community. Thus, it is always possible to ask of a statement appearing in a professional code: Even though the professional group agrees that a given behavior is ethically appropriate, it is really consistent with the basic principles of our ethical system? The code itself can never be taken by a society as the ultimate test of the morality of a lay-professional rolationohip. A full cthicol onolysis of the iole of physicians in for-profit health care enterprise must include an examination of the basic ethical issues, not merely an effort to determine what the professional code writers believe to be ethical.

Basic Philosophical Themes

Business Ethics and Physician Ethics: The Role of Altruism   The most fundamental ethical issue arising when the physician confronts the world of business is whether the ethic of the physician is compatible with that of the business world. It has been argued that the ethical obligations that define the role of the physician are derived from basic ethical principles shared by the moral community of lay persons and professionals. Thus, in principle the ethics of business and the ethics of a profession should have a common foundation. Different individual roles in a society, however, may require radically different moral actions even though the moral obligations defining those roles are all derived from a common set of principles. Parents, teachers, and police officers ought to treat adolescents differently even though they all subscribe to the same system of ethical principles. Likewise, it may be that business people and physicians ought to act somewhat differently toward clients even though they subscribe to the same general principles.

A commonly held stereotype that expresses such differences is that physicians and other health care professionals are expected to act primarily or exclusively for the welfare of the patient, whereas it is perfectly acceptable for an ordinary business person to pursue self-interest even at the expense of the welfare of others. In the literature on the sociology of the professions, professionals are distinguished from occupations by what Talcott Parsons called "collectivity orientation."[37] That is, they pursue interests common to the group rather than just self-interest. It is what in ethics would be referred to as altruism rather than egoism. By contrast business persons are self-oriented or egoistic; they are not expected to put the welfare of others above or even on the same plane as their own interests. It is not that business people are being selfish and immoral. Rather, it is considered ethically appropriate for the business person to pursue self-interest when in the business role. As long as that fundamental ethical distinction holds, it is apparent that it will be extremely difficult for the health care professional's role to be embedded a business context. When professionals are employees of profit-making corporations, pursuing their role predictably would clash with business persons within the corporation pursuing theirs. When professionals are themselves owners of for-profit health care enterprises, they would themselves experience the conflict of trying to fill the two roles simultaneously.

There is good evidence, however, that the distinction between self- and collectivity orientation is overstated and much too simplistic. It has already been pointed out that health care professionals themselves are increasingly recognizing the legitimacy of a muted self-interest in their ethics. On the other hand, it is clear that the ethic of business has never been one in which anything goes as long as self-interest is served. It is safe to say that virtually no business person believes that business people should lie, cheat, steal, or harm others. (Of course, in the world of business, just as in the world of professions, no one always conforms perfectly to the norm of what should be done.) Business people see themselves as having many characteristics in common with professionals, including the recognition of moral limits on pursuit of self-interest. Physicians, on the other hand, increasingly see themselves as having elements in common with business persons, including a degree of legitimate self-interest.

This is not to say that the ethical norms for physicians and for business people are identical. It is clear they are not. The difference cannot be reduced simplistically, however, to a difference between self- and collectivity orientations.

What is as stake may be the extent to which society expects people in each role to be altruistic. It may be that certain limited acts of kindness and other-regarding actions are expected of the business community. Business people widely follow the practice of making charitable contributions and engaging in other beneficent actions, not all of which can be attributed to enlightened self-interest. These, especially if they involve substantial contribution, are typically viewed as supererogatory, as acts above and beyond what strict morality requires.

On the other hand, although the codes of physicians contain platitudes about the welfare of the patient always taking absolute moral precedence, physicians recognize that there are legitimate moral limits on the obligation to sacrifice self-interest for the welfare of others. Virtually no study has been made within the ethics of professions to examine the real moral limits on the professional's duty to be collectivity oriented or on the relation between the professional's obligation to be altruistic in comparison with the business person's.

Deontological versus Consequentialist Ethics   Another potential but unexplored difference between professional and business ethics may bo found in the technical distinction made by philosophical ethicists between deontological and consequentialist modes of reasoning. It is now well established that physicians, in their traditional professional ethics, are uniquely consequentialist in their moral reasoning. They evaluate actions strictly on the basis of the consequences they produce. Physician ethics is even more unique in that in comparison to, say, public policy analysts, many of whom also are consequentialist in their ethics, the relevant consequences for physicians are limited, at least in the classical expressions of the Hippocratic tradition, to those accruing to patients (rather than to other individuals, bystanders, or society at large). Thus, this consequentialist thinking differs from classical utilitarianism.

To this author's knowledge, no thorough study of the normative ethical structure of the business community has ever been undertaken. I would predict, however, that although the business ethic is not immune from consequentialist thinking, especially of the utilitarian type, it is much closer to the traditional religious ethics (especially Jewish and Protestant ethics) and the secular liberal tradition of our political and cultural heritage (stemming from natural law theory, Locke, Hobbes, Kant, and the American founding fathers). As different as these traditions are, they all share a common feature: They all maintain that there is more to ethics than simply producing good consequences. Lying, breaking promises, violating the liberty of others, and killing are characteristics of actions that tend to make them wrong even if in a particular instance bad consequences do not flow from those actions. This position is what ethicists call deontological ethics. A brief examination of the codes of the business community reveals tendencies to display that kind of reasoning in addition to utilitarian patterns. Business people think it is wrong to lie, cheat, and steal, and they do not have to determine the consequences before they reach that conclusion. If so, they are very different from physicians in their traditional consequentialist ethical theory.

Health Care as a Commodity   One possibility is that the difference between business and professional ethics is not in the roles of the participants but in the nature of the "product." It is currently being debated heatedly whether health care is unique among the goods and services in which people potentially have an interest. On the one hand, some argue that health care is like any other commodity—like beer or panty hose, to use the language of one who takes this position. It should be sold in the market to those who have the capacity to buy. After all, it is pointed out, such other basic necessities as food, clothing, and shelter are sold similarly. This is the position of the libertarians, under the influence of entitlement theorists,[38] and of health care theorists under that sphere of influence.[39] From such a philosophical perspective, it is easy to see how health care could become part of for-profit corporate enterprise without any moral tensions.

On the other hand, some see health care as more fundamental. While it is recognized that people cannot have an unlimited right to all the health care they could possibly want, health care is viewed as different from other goods and services, something to which one has some kind of moral right. It is viewed that way because it is fundamental to survival, because the need for it is distributed so unevenly, or because it is necessary to enjoy the basic social goods of life.[40] It is a position rooted in more patterned theories of distributive justice.[41]

The implications are radical if one views health care as some sort of right and thus different from mere business commodities. It makes the delivery of health care in a business setting almost impossible. The implications extend far beyond corporate for-profit enterprises of the kind that are beginning to emerge on the American scene. All distribution of health care on an economic basis is called into question, even the more traditional professional private-practitioner/fee-for-service arrangements. The profit motive itself, which we have seen to be compatible with traditional professional physician ethics, is jeopardized in the health care sphere if health care is a right.

The Double Agent Problem   Another basic theme that makes the business/health care relationship unique is what has been referred to by medical ethicists over the past decade as the double agent problem. As we have seen, many business/professional relationships involve relatively simple diadic interactions in which the professional is engaged by the corporation to serve the corporation's interest. The lawyer or engineer performs the services needed by the corporation. In relatively rare circumstances the professional is hired by the organization to provide professional services directly for a client who may have interests quite different from the organization's. The professional is simultaneously an agent for the organization and an individual client. The term *double agent problem* was first used to describe the position of a psychiatrist employed by a medical school to provide psychiatric services to medical students but who was also to advise the school on the suitability of students for continuation or reentry into its educational program.[42]

A physician employed by a corporation who would sell his or her services to customers of the corporation is potentially in the classical doublo agcnt bind. Loyalty to the corporation may conflict with that which is traditionally owed to the patient. It is not yet clear what the proper ethical dynamic should be for a professional in a double agent situation. Some argue that professionals simply cannot function in such a situation. That would mean that no physician should be working for a profit-making corporation if the agenda were potentially in conflict with that of patients (which it always would be).

Most now consider that answer too simple. In at least some carefully guarded contexts health care professionals are thought to be acting ethically while having divided loyalties. Company physicians offering employment physical exams, for example, are widely accepted. The strategy that is evolving is one of developing principles for reducing or eliminating conflict of interest. For example, principles of disclosure are being formulated. All parties should know in advance exactly what kinds of information should be disclosed to employers and what to keep confidential. If physicians in a corporate setting are expected to make cost containment decisions whereby patients might not receive all the care that was potentially beneficial to them, at the very least the physician would be expected to disclose to all parties that such decisions were part of his or her role. It is unlikely, however, that full disclosure alone will solve the double agent problem. As the practice of medicine in a for-profit enterprise evolves, a study of additional safeguards and guidelines to minimize conflict of interest must be developed.

Differences Between Business and Physician Ethics

It has been argued that it is too simple to distinguish between the ethics of the physician and the business person by holding that physicians, as professionals, are collectively oriented and business people are self-oriented. Still it was held that there are differences in traditional ethical expectations in the two roles. In this section several of the more specific examples of these conflicts will be presented, based on a review of the literature of business and professional ethics and general knowledge of traditional patterns and beliefs. It is suggested that these more specific ethical problems will likely constitute the heart of the ethical tension between business and professional models if and when the practice of medicine in a for-profit setting becomes dominant.

Lying and Deception Before turning to several examples of direct relevance to health care economics, it is interesting to note one example of ethical differences between health care professionals and business people that supports the claim that the ethical differences are more complex than the common stereotype would admit. It is fair to say that there is nothing in business ethics that requires telling the "whole truth" about one's product. Certain disclosures are surely required, but the weak points or inadequacies of one's product need not be emphasized. Still an outright lie misrepresenting one's product, claiming that it has some property that it does not have, is ethically unacceptable in the business community. (Again, this is not to say it does not happen, but when it does no one in the business community is going to defend the lie as morally acceptable).

By contrast, in professional physician ethics the dominant moral principle has been the welfare of the patient. Deception, misinformation, and outright lies have been defended morally when done in the name of protecting patient welfare—to avoid traumatizing a terminal cancer patient or to entice a patient into needed medical treatment. The professional ethical evaluation of this practice has changed rapidly over the past decade.[43] Such deception is now widely rejected among physicians. The newest version of the Principles of Medical Ethics of the AMA holds the physician to "deal honestly with patients." That is a new recognition of the rights of patients. Prior to these recent developments, however, physicians and business people had clear differences on the morality of lying—differences, oddly enough, in which the business person held a position closer to traditional Western morality.

Competitor's Use of Outdated Information   The remaining differences that will be identified between physician morality and business morality relate directly to tensions one can anticipate in the evolution of the practice of medicine in for-profit corporate settings. Consider, as a first example, a situation in which a practitioner discovers that a competitor is making business decisions based on outdated, erroneous, or inadequate information. If that individual is in the business world, this is likely to be a cause for rejoicing. Nothing in the ethics of business would call for that business person to point this fact out to his competitor. In fact, he or she would be expected to take advantage of it to improve the market position of the business.

A physician discovering that a colleague is using outdated, erroneous, or inadequate information is morally in a very different position. Such a physician bears an obligation to take reasonable steps to enlighten the colleague, transmit up-to-date information, and if necessary even take action to make sure that the colleague practices competently. The difference in the relation is signaled by the shift in language from competitor to colleague. A physician who works for one profit-making corporation and who learns that a colleague who works for a competing hospital is using an outmoded practice that will eventually be disadvantageous to his or her employer as well as the patients would find it difficult at best to fulfill simultaneously the traditional ethical expectations of both business and professional medicine.

Enticement of Customers into Needless Consumption   Another area of potential tension is in practices that entice customers to consume. It is widely accepted in business through advertising, packaging, and other promotion techniques that it is not only ethical but also necessary business strategy to create a market for one's product. A good profit-oriented hospital should be expected to do just that—by promoting elective procedures; making efficient use of resources; and encouraging or giving incentives to physicians to "order" marginal tests, treatments, and services. Although business people probably would find unacceptable the intentional inducement of a consumer to use a product that would actually be harmful, little objection is ever offered to harmless enticement to consume.

In medicine the traditional pattern is quite different. Although physicians may engage in practices that serve only to generate extra business for them, such practices are certainly considered unethical. In the extreme, such as in Medicaid "mills," universal condemnation is the response. Once one realizes that many procedures, tests, and treatments are quite marginal—that a patient will neither be helped nor hurt greatly by an intervention—the problem becomes more critical. Physicians can expect to come under great pressure from corporate managers to generate work in these areas.

Exclusion of Inefficient Customers   Another common, prudent business practice is the exclusion of customers who can only be serviced inefficiently. If a company services a large market, one portion of which is sparsely populated and is being serviced at a loss, a corporate executive would be viewed as foolish—perhaps even unethical in squandering stockholders' resources—were he or she to fail to close the territory that placed a drain on the company.

In medicine efforts to exclude service to areas and individuals who can be served only at relatively great cost are much more suspect. The closing of a rural clinic or a government decision to transfer public health service personnel away from sparsely settled areas would certainly meet with controversy. For-profit health care corporations providing hospital care are certain to face conflict over these divergent patterns of expectation. The morally correct solution to this dilemma probably will depend directly on whether health care is a right or a mere commodity.

The Duty to the Indigent   Another dilemma closely related to the question of whether health care is a right is what business people and physicians feel they owe to those who cannot afford to purchase services at the prevailing market rate. No business person would think that he or she has a duty to provide a Mercedes or even a Ford to those who cannot afford to buy one, but physicians traditionally have held some sense of responsibility to those too poor to buy medical care. Physicians have acknowledged both charity work and the principle of the sliding-scale fee. Although sometimes these are acknowledged more in theory than in practice (one study in Connecticut revealed that no analytical psychiatrist treated patients for free, though there were limited cases of fee reduction),[44] some sense of responsibility, collective or individual, is still acknowledged. Hospitals receiving Hill-Burton funds are obligated by law to offer services to the indigent. It is predictable that physicians will feel tension with their corporate employers when indigent patients arrive at the hospital door needing unaffordable medical services.

Supplying Unprofitable Products and Services   One of the great problems faced by the business model, especially if health care is considered a right of more rigorous claim than mere commodities, is how goods and services that lack profit potential will ever be produced. We already face that problem with the production of drugs and biologicals for rare conditions in which commercial production can never be profitable. Similar problems exist potentially for goods and services in hospitals and other commercially owned health care facilities. The development of surgeons trained to perform rarely needed surgical procedures could probably never take place in a purely market model. Certain types of medical interventions are more easily provided for a fee than others. Some concern has already been expressed that drug, surgical, and other treatment interventions will be overemphasized at the expense of dietary and lifestyle changes because it is difficult to collect as lucrative a fee for counseling as for more tangible services. Any intervention strategy that however effective lacks profit potential may be jeopardized in the for-profit enterprise system of health care delivery.

Of course, these problems have been faced already. Some drug companies conduct important work on pharmaceuticals that they know lack profit potential. They do so for the public relations value but probably also out of a limited sense of altruism. Moreover, the government carries a substantial portion of the burden for research and development in areas for which the profit incentive is inadequate. If for-profit health care enterprise becomes more widespread, it may have to be supplemented by a governmental support network for research, development, and delivery of products and services lacking profit potential.

Differing Concepts of Self-Regulation   One of the chief characteristics of a profession well recognized by the sociology of the professions is that professionals, as opposed to those merely engaged in business, have substantial authority for self-regulation. This is expressed in a professional role in licensure, certification, supervision of curriculum, disciplinary proceedings, and accreditation. By contrast, the business world basically has been exempt from efforts of self-regulation. Voluntary efforts have been weak, reliant on moral suasion, and widely regarded as ineffective.

There are both theoretical and practical reasons professional self-regulation in these areas has come under severe criticism. In theory, if professional groups have unique ethical and other value commitments, then even perfect self-regulation will sometimes produce results that are unacceptable to the broader community. On the practical level it is widely recognized that the pressures of conflict of interest and comradeship make effective self-regulation extremely difficult. Thus, there is strong pressure for society to treat the professions more like businesses, with a combination of internal voluntary efforts, regulatory restraint, judicial control, and public accountability. Still we can anticipate potential tension, for example, when physicians in a commercially owned hospital feel accountable to outsiders within their profession and the business managers resist professional efforts to control their business practices.

Conclusion

We can anticipate many points of ethical difficulty as for-profit health care enterprises evolve and force more direct interactions between the medical profession and its system of ethics and business with its system of ethics. It is not yet clear what the organized professional physician response will be to these developments. We can anticipate that physicians will be concerned with any removal of professional control from medical decision making and will be uncomfortable with the assault on their dignity that would accompany an increase in the image of commercialization of the physician's role. Still we have repeatedly seen the organized profession accommodate change by moving in the direction of the business model. Shifts on advertising, accommodation to ownership of health facilities, repeated endorsements of the legitimacy of the profit motive, and adjustments to tolerate the employment of the professional within lay organizations all point to the flexibility of the profession on such matters and its ability to accommodate the realities of health care as an industry.

It is not clear what the public ought to say regarding the practice of medicine in a for-profit commercial setting. An initial intuitive resistance to it is grounded in the traditional high regard for the medical professional, an unwillingness to view the physician as part of a business operation, and a feeling that health care should be supplied (within some reasonable limits) on the basis of need rather than ability to pay. If the debate over whether all of health care should be insulated from the market of supply and demand leads to the conclusion that it should be, then public resistance to medicine within a for-profit enterprise would be expected.

On the other hand, the case can be made for a further opening toward the practice of medicine in this way. Many of the recent changes in professional physician ethics—the development of the rights perspective, the movement away from an exclusively consequentialist ethic, and the acceptance of the legitimacy of a limited self-interest—stem from lay pressures on the professional community to return to the mainstream of Western ethics. Physicians and lay people alike may find attractive a liberation from the unreasonable expectation of unlimited altruism on the part of physicians. Such an adjustment would make the lay-professional relationship a more realistic one of equal human beings, each of whom has something to gain from an interaction. Moreover, if our society is moving away from professional self-regulation and toward more public mechanisms of control comparable to those now in place in the business community, the evolution of a for-profit commercial medical system might facilitate that shift.

The time has come to explore in much greater depth the ethical tensions that will arise as for-profit health care systems controlled by nonprofessional business interests begin to gain a greater position in our society. Study is needed both of the more theoretical differences between professional and business ethics and the specific ethical problems that are likely to arise.

References and Notes

1. The early seventeenth-century figure, Kunh T'ing-hsein, complained of the physicians who were his contemporaries: "When they visit the rich, they are conscientious; when they deal with the poor, they act carelessly. This is the eternal peculiarity of those who practice medicine as a profession, and not as applied humaneness." Cited in Paul U. Unschuld, *Medical Ethics in Imperial China* (Berkeley: University of California Press, 1979), p. 74.

2. Darrel W. Amundsen, "The Physician's Obligation to Prolong Life: A Medical Duty Without Classical Roots," *Hastings Center Report* 8 (August 1978), pp. 23-30.

3. Galen, De Placitis 9, 5, as cited in Darrel W. Amundsen, op. cit., p. 24.

4. Thomas Percival, *Percival's Medical Ethics*, edited by Chauncey D. Leake (Baltimore: Williams & Wilkins, 1927).

5. British Medical Association, *Medical Ethics* (London: British Medical Association House, 1974).

6. The Australian Code informed the physician that: "A doctor should not have a financial interest in the sale of any pharmaceutical preparation that he may recommend to a patient. . . ." But at the same time, "this is not held to apply to the acquisition of shares in a public company marketing pharmaceutical products, subject to the provision that the acquisition of shares is not conditional on ordering products of the company. . . ." Australian Medical Association, *Code of Ethics* (Glebe, Sidney: Australian Medical Association, 1975 edition), p. 24.

7. American Medical Association, *Code of Medical Ethics*, adopted by the AMA in Philadelphia, May 1847, and by the New York Academy of Medicine in October 1847 (New York: H. Ludwig & Co., 1848), p. 17.

8. "Principles of Medical Ethics of the American Medical Association," 1903, 1912. Reprinted in *Percival's Medical Ethics*, op. cit. pp. 244, 260.

9. American Medical Association, *Judicial Council and Reports* (Chicago: American Medical Association, 1971), p. 23.

10. American Medical Association, *Code of Medical Ethics*, adopted by the AMA at Philadelphia, May 1847, and by the New York Academy of Medicine in October 1847 (New York: H. Ludwig, & Co., 1848), p. 17.

11. "It is not unethical for a physician to patent a surgical or diagnostic instrument . . . but in the interest of the public welfare and the dignity of the profession [medicine] insists that once a patent is obtained by a physician . . . the physician may not ethically use his patent right to retard or inhibit research or to restrict the benefit derivable from the patented article. Any physician who obtains a patent and uses it for his own aggrandizement or financial interest to the detriment of the profession or the public is acting unethically." *Judicial Council Opinions and Reports* (Chicago: American Medical Association, 1971), p. 13.

12. In fact it is gratuitously added that: "The laws governing patents are based on the sound doctrine that one is entitled to protect his discovery." *Current Opinions of the Judicial Council of the American Medical Association* (Chicago: American Medical Association, 1981), p. 29.

13. "If such nostrum be of real efficacy," says the 1847 code, "any concealment regarding it is inconsistent with benefidence and professional liberality; and, if mystery alone give it value and importance, such craft implies either disgraceful ignorance, or fraudulent avarice." *Code of Medical Ethics*, adopted by the American Medical Association at Philadelphia, May 1847, and by the New York Academy of Medicine in October 1847 (New York: H. Ludwig & Co., 1848), p. 17.

14. American Medical Association, *Judicial Council Opinions and Reports* (Chicago: American Medical Association, 1971), pp. 37, 48.

15. Ibid., p. 48.

16. Ibid., p. 41; *Current Opinions of the Judicial Council of the American Medical Association* (Chicago: American Medical Association, 1981), p. 20.

17. "Report of the Judicial Council of the American Medical Association." *Journal of the American Medical Association* 134 (May 10, 1947), p. 178.

18. *Judicial Council Opinions and Reports* (Chicago: American Medical Association, 1971), p. 37.

19. Mark V. Pauly, "The Ethics and Economics of Kickbacks and Fee Splitting," *Bell Journal of Economics* 10 (September 1979), pp. 334-352.

20. *Current Opinions of the Judicial Council of the American Medical Association* (Chicago: American Medical Association, 1971), p. 24.

21. Ibid., p. 11.

22. Ibid.

23. Ibid., pp. 25-26.

24. *Judicial Council Opinions and Reports* (Chicago: American Medical Association, 1977), p. 39.

25. *Judicial Council Opinion and Reports* (Chicago: American Medical Association, 1969), pp. 32-35; *Judicial Council Opinions and Reports* (Chicago: American Medical Association, 1971), pp. 31-33.

26. *Judicial Council Opinion and Reports* (Chicago: American Medical Association, 1969), p. 32.

27. Ibid., pp. 32-33.

28. Paul U. Unschuld, *Medical Ethics in Imperial China* (Berkeley: University of California Press, 1979).

29. Speaking of the physician's relation with laboratories, it said: "As a professional man, the physician is entitled to fair compensation for his services. He is not engaged in a commercial enterprise and he should not make a markup, commission, or profit on the services rendered by others." *Current Opinions of the Judicial Council of the American Medical Association* (Chicago: American Medical Association, 1981), p. 26.

30. Robert M. Veatch, *Case Studies in Medical Ethics* (Cambridge: Harvard University Press, 1977), pp. 61-64.

31. Jane Clapp, *Professional Ethics and Insignia* (Metuchen, N.J.: Scarecrow Press, Inc., 1974), p. 9.

32. Ibid., pp. 247-248.

33. Clarence Walton, *The Ethics of Corporate Conduct* (Englewood Cliffs, N.J.: Prentice-Hall, 1977), pp. 305-338.

34. "The professional services of a lawyer should not be controlled or exploited by any lay agency, personal or corporate, which intervenes between the client and lawyer." Henry S. Drinker, *Legal Ethics* (Westport, Conn.: Greenwood Press, 1980), p. 322.

35. Ibid. Employment in an organization, such as an association, club, or trade organization, was acceptable provided the lawyer rendered legal services to that organization, "but this employment should not include the rendering of legal services to the members of such an organization in respect to their individual affairs."

36. *Recent Ethics Opinions: Committee on Ethics and Professional Responsibility* (Chicago: American Bar Association, from March 1969 to July 1976).

37. Talcott Parsons, *The Social System* (New York: The Free Press, 1951), p. 434.

38. Robert Nozick, *Anarchy, State and Utopia* (New York: Basic Books, 1974).

39. H. Tristram Engelhardt, Jr., "Health Care Allocations: Response to the Unjust, the Unfortunate, and the Undesirable," In Earl Shelp, ed. *Justice and Health Care* (Dordrecht, Holland: D. Reidel Publishing Co., 1981), pp. 121-137.

40. Ronald Green, "Health Care and Justice in Contract Theory Perspective," Robert M. Veatch and Roy Branson, eds. *Ethics and Health Policy* (Cambridge: Ballinger, 1976), pp. 111-126.; Gene Outka, "Social Justice and Equal Access to Health Care," *Journal of Religious Ethics* 2 (Spring 1974), pp. 11-32; Robert M. Veatch, *A Theory of Medical Ethics* (New York: Basic Books, 1981), pp. 250-287.

41. John Rawls, *A Theory of Justice* (Cambridge: Harvard University Press, 1971); Christopher Abe, "Justice as Equality," *Philosophy and Public Affairs* 5 (Fall 1975), pp. 69-89.

42. Willard Gaylin and Daniel Callahan, "The Psychiatrist as Double Agent," *Hastings Center Report* 4 (February 1974), pp. 12-14.

43. Robert M. Veatch and Ernest Tai, "Talking About Death: Patterns of Lay and Professional Change," *Annals of the American Academy of Political and Social Science* 447 (January 1980), pp. 29-45.

44. August Hollingshead and Fredrick C. Redlich, *Social Class and Mental Illness: A Community Study* (New York: John Wiley & Sons, 1966, reprint of 1958 edition), p. 314.

Secondary Income From Recommended Treatment: Should Fiduciary Principles Constrain Physician Behavior?

Frances H. Miller

It is generally recognized that the parties to a physician-patient relationship are frequently on unequal footing. The potential for physician dominance stems not only from the fact that illness places patients in a vulnerable, dependent posture but also from the superior knowledge, training, and clinical experience of the physician. Although it may be difficult for the average patient to question the physician's judgment, patients must lay their innermost selves bare, both physically and emotionally, if their doctors are to understand the true nature and origin of their problems. Without trust, and therefore vulnerability, the candor necessary to the therapeutic relationship is impossible to achieve.

The law redresses this kind of imbalance in certain relationships by requiring people who occupy positions of trust, such as physicians, to subordinate self-interest to the well-being of their charges. Such a relationship is called a fiduciary relationship. A fiduciary—from the Latin *fides*, meaning trust, fidelity, or confidence—is a person who occupies a position of trust, fidelity, or confidence in relation to someone else. The physician's conduct is not measured by that of, for example, the used-car salesman, because the principle of *caveat emptor* appropriate to arm's-length bargaining has no place in the doctor-patient relationship.

As fiduciaries, doctors owe a duty of loyalty to their patient's interests that requires them to elevate their conduct above that of commercial actors. In the words of Mr. Justice Cardozo:

Many forms of conduct permissible in a workaday world for those acting at arm's
length, are forbidden to those bound by fiduciary ties. A . . . [fiduciary] is held to
something stricter than the morals of the market place. Not honesty alone, but
the punctilio of an honor the most sensitive, is then the standard of behavior.[1]

The potential for conflict of interest, and therefore abuse of trust, is
ordinarily what brings fiduciary principles into play, but conflict of
interest in fact is not essential to fiduciary status.

This paper describes the law's current approach to fiduciary aspects
of physician-patient interaction. In tracing the development of the
concept, issues have been analyzed for their potential impact on physician involvement in profit-making medical enterprises. A broad perspective was deemed useful to understand the subtle way in which
fiduciary notions surround the physician-patient relationship with
constraints on behavior not found in ordinary commercial transactions. Those constraints in turn are relevant to physician participation
in what Dr. Arnold Relman has termed the medical-industrial complex,[2] even though they may have arisen in an entirely different context. On the basis of an analysis of fiduciary theory, this paper concludes
that a physician's receipt of secondary income from the treatment he
or she advises for a patient raises the spectre of wrongful manipulation
of the trust essential to the physician-patient relationship.

The Physician-Patient Conflict of Interest Problem

At a fundamental level a patient's best interests will not always coincide with what seems to be the physician's most advantageous financial or professional position. Physicians are uniquely situated to
persuade patients to purchase medical services, for patients rarely
possess the sophisticated diagnostic skills that would prompt them to
second guess physician advice. Moreover, when physicians are paid
on a fee-for-service basis, their income increases the more services
they provide, regardless of whether the patient actually needs them.
If the physician works for a profit-sharing independent practice association (IPA) or health maintenance organization (HMO), the fewer
services he or she provides the more money the physician makes at
the end of the year, because patients pay by capitation. Similarly, the
less time physicians on salary spend with patients, the more time they
have for other professional pursuits. In these last two situations pa-

tients may not suspect they are getting short shrift because of the trust inherent in the physician-patient relationship. The threat of malpractice litigation helps to keep these incentives to over- and underuse medical care within bounds, but the possibility of conflict of interest at this primary level is inevitable because of one or another of these economic incentives.[3]

A different kind of conflict of interest, which could in large part be avoided, is involved when physicians derive secondary income from the care they order for their patients. This happens whenever physicians own substantial equity interests in medical service organizations to which they refer patients.[4] Physician owners or shareholders in a hospital or nursing home do not realize their full income potential when the facility's beds are not fully occupied. When they can fill empty beds with their own patients, the economic incentive to inappropriate use is obvious. Likewise, a physician with a substantial financial interest in a laboratory, a CAT scanner, or a home health care service usually profits in direct relation to the number of lab tests, CAT scans, or paraprofessional services performed. The temptation for a doctor-owner to prescribe excessive quantities of these items is undeniable. They are usually covered by insurance; thus, reimbursement is certain and the patient does not pay directly out-of-pocket for their cost.

More disturbing, physician-owners of dialysis centers have sometimes been suspected of placing their renal patients on dialysis sooner than necessary to keep their profit-making stations fully used. Some have been accused of dragging their heels on the question of kidney transplants, which might obviate the need for dialysis altogether. Their bias against home dialysis, which is cheaper to deliver but arguably more risky, also has been noted. Because the original projections of how much it would cost to cover dialysis under Medicare were so wide of the mark,[5] there has been much speculation about how much, if any, of the increase in cost can be attributed to the fact that a high percentage of dialysis is delivered by for-profit providers.[6] The dual capacity in which physician-owners of dialysis facilities function lends a credibility to this concern that would be diminished in direct proportion to the degree of separation between their diagnostic and therapeutic roles.

In all of these cases of physician involvement in for-profit medicine the conflict of interest could be avoided without damaging the essence of the physician-patient relationship. Simply prohibiting physicians from functioning in a dual capacity with respect to their patients would suffice. Physicians need not be forbidden to own nursing homes ur dialysis facilities. Rather, they would not be allowed to send their own patients there. There are obvious disadvantages to such a solution because, for example, physicians might pay more attention to maintaining the standards of a nursing home if their patients resided there. There are also ways to circumvent it, because physicians could simply agree to send their patients to each other's profit-making facilities. However, other methods of enforcing standards and discouraging collusive behavior exist, and a prohibition at least would do away with the direct incentive to prescribe inappropriate care.

The real question is whether such a remedy is necessary or whether mere disclosure of the conflict of interest would sufficiently eliminate the potential for abuse. Is any "remedy" at all even appropriate? Alternatively, does physician involvement in for-profit medical care pose such a threat that more drastic responses are in order? The answers to these questions are unavoidably complex. They are also beyond the scope of this paper, because the true magnitude of abuse is difficult to gauge on the basis of available information. A discussion of how the law treats the fiduciary aspects of the physician-patient relationship, however, might throw some light on the issues.

Background of Fiduciary Law

Determining when a fiduciary relationship exists and exactly what standard of conduct applies is no easy task. The term *fiduciary* has been called "one of the most ill-defined, if not altogether misleading terms in . . . law."[7] Courts have deliberately refrained from precisely defining the nature of fiduciary duty, on the theory that they need flexibility to deal with the innumerable permutations of relationships and behavior spawned by changing economic and social conditions.

Fiduciary remedies originally sprang from courts of equity rather than courts of law, because the law provided no redress for breaches of trust.[8] The label "fiduciary" need not necessarily be reserved for situations in which equitable rather than legal relief is requested, but the standard of care governing recovery in certain kinds of common law actions, such as for medical malpractice, may be heavily influenced by professional ethics with an "equity" origin. Fiduciary terminology thus appears in cases that allege violation of ordinary legal duty as well as less well defined fiduciary obligation. Courts also tend to use fiduciary terminology loosely to bolster a "correct" policy result when the factual circumstances support recovery for the plaintiff without the added moral weight of separate fiduciary concepts. Generally speaking, the law seems to affix the fiduciary label to specific factual situations, rather than to be guided by a well-structured theory of fiduciary obligation against which particular behavior can be tested. Analysis of the fiduciary aspects of physician-patient relationships thus is hindered by the lack of a precise analytical framework within which to examine the issue.

Fiduciary Theory in Medical Litigation

There are certain basic principles that help place the physician-as-fiduciary problem in perspective. Fiduciary relationships usually fall into one of three general categories—with the fiduciary seen as (1) guardian of property, (2) advisor, or (3) agent.[9] The law may impose fiduciary responsibilities on physicians stemming from more than one of these categories. The following sections discuss cases in the context of these categories and speculate on the way they might apply to physicians' receipt of secondary income as a result of their treatment recommendations.

Physician as Guardian of Patient Property

The first category of fiduciary relationships applies to persons entrusted with other people's property. They are required to deal with the property so as to enhance the interests of their beneficiaries, even if that comes at the expense of their own interests. A trustee, for example, may not self-deal with respect to trust assets. If a trustee does, no matter how objectively reasonable the transaction may appear, any benefit to the trustee will inure to the trust and any loss must be made up from the trustee's own pocket.

Although physicians ordinarily have no direct control over their patients' property, they do have enormous power over the medical costs their patients incur. To the extent that financial self-interest—particularly in the secondary income sense—has the tendency to skew their medical advice, physicians may be considered fiduciaries with respect to their patients' financial resources.

Kickback Cases   Courts have not hesitated to condemn practices whereby physicians accept kickbacks for breach of fiduciary obligation to their patients. Thus, when a physician agreed with a lawyer to refer personal injury claimants in return for a kickback equal to the difference between the medical bill and one half of the combined medical and legal fees, the Massachusetts Supreme Judicial Court was characteristically acerbic in finding that the state licensing board had jurisdiction to revoke his license. Noting the physician's "high moral duty" to serve patients before he served himself, the court commented that "very few . . . patients would be pleased to know that . . . [their doctor] had received in addition to his medical bill a further sum out of the patient's money for no service rendered to the patient."[10]

Similarly, a federal Court of Appeals strongly condemned the practice whereby optical companies kicked back one-third of the retail price of eyeglasses to referring eye specialists. Labeling the arrangements as "unconscionable and reprehensible contracts for secret kickbacks to a doctor," the court specifically found that they corrupted the fiduciary relationship between physician and patient.[11] Not only do kickbacks distort a physician's incentive for referral from its proper focus—the best interests of the patient—but they also inflate the cost of the referred product or service. To the extent that the second provider builds the cost of the kickback into the cost of the referred item, its price goes up unnecessarily. Recent allegations of corrupt sales practices in the cardiac pacemaker industry provide a dramatic illustration of the inflationary impact of kickbacks.[12]

These cases bear as strongly on patient financial well-being as they do on patient physical health.[13] The courts' opinions focus on the way the doctors' breaches of fiduciary duty impaired their patients' property interests by forcing them to pay unnecessary costs. If one applies this logic to the situation of physician involvement in for-profit medicine, the parallels at first seem close. In fact, physician involvement in profit-making medical enterprises looks even worse because the "kickbacks," or secondary income, actually come from the physicians themselves in their corporate *persona*. On closer examination, however, the factor that artificially inflates costs in the kickback cases— the fee for merely "referring"—is absent. Costs may be just as artificially inflated if the care is unnecessary, but this will not be the case universally. (The same concerns arise when the kickback is more sophisticated and less visible in the nonprofit context, as when physicians with high volumes of hospital admissions are rewarded with nominal or nonexistent rental charges for office space in hospital-owned buildings.) The kickback opinions suggest that disclosure of the conflict of interest might obviate the breach of fiduciary duty, and disclosure of the receipt of secondary income from recommended treatment options might go a long way toward alleviating the potential for abuse associated with physician ownership of the business entities to which he or she makes referrals.

Reimbursement Cases   There is another sense, however, in which physicians may be considered fiduciaries with respect to their patients' property. It is sometimes argued that a physician has a fiduciary obligation to the patient's pocketbook when it comes to prescribing medical care.[14] The practice of hospitalizing patients for treatments that could be provided less expensively on an outpatient basis but that are covered by insurance only if done on inpatients is consistent with that thesis. The Robin Hood method of pricing widely practiced by physicians prior to the advent of Medicare and Medicaid—subsidizing medical care for the poor by surcharging the rich—is a variation on the same theme. The physician's fiduciary role in both of these situations involves the patient's finances in addition to his or her health. Whether the law imposes such a fiduciary responsibility on physicians, however, is virtually untested in the courts.

Occasionally a patient will seek to recover from the physician the cost of hospitalization that was determined to be unnecessary, and therefore unreimbursable, by a third-party payor's retrospective utilization review procedure. Those few cases may mention fiduciary principles in passing, but the theory for allowing the patient to recover hospital costs from the physician is usually breach of an implied contract not to prescribe unnecessary care. The potential for expansion of fiduciary liability in this area exists, however. Physicians clearly know better than patients when care is medically unnecessary and therefore vulnerable to an insurer's claims rejection process. In addition, they usually have a fairly clear idea about what kinds of care are likely to be reimbursable. A medically unsophisticated patient, on the other hand, ordinarily is reluctant to question a physician's opinion that he or she be hospitalized or undergo certain forms of therapy. Notwithstanding the rhetoric about informed consent, patients are conditioned to defer to physicians on matters of medical judgment. The analogy to trust law, although not perfect, is thus apt. The physician could be viewed as a trustee of the patient's financial resources, including insurance, with a fiduciary obligation to consider both health and finances in using them in the patient's best interests.

If physicians are considered such *de facto* trustees, when they derive secondary income from the treatment prescribed for their patients, they are in effect self-dealing. As previously noted, however, the law protects trust beneficiaries by prohibiting a trustee from benefiting by self-dealing. The temptations for abuse are considered so overwhelming that courts have responded by effectively eliminating any opportunity for gain on the part of the trustee. If one were to accept the trust analogy as appropriately applied to physician ownership of health care organizations, one would have to insulate physicians from any secondary income generated by their medical advice.

Gift and Contract Cases   Gift and contract cases involving physicians and patients fit neatly into the lay understanding of fiduciary transactions, for they seek direct recovery of the patient's property or to nullify the patient's contractual obligations. The kickback and reimbursement opinions also concern the patient's property rights, but in a more subtle sense. In those situations health insurance may have blunted the patient's awareness of the financial impact of receiving artificially costly or unnecessary care.

The theory underlying the gift and contract cases involves the potential for undue influence generated by the physician's dominant position in the relationship.[15] These cases concern the physician's fiduciary role with respect to patient property rather than patient health. The fact that the fiduciary happens to be a physician is incidental to the analysis. It could just as well be a lawyer, a stockbroker, or anyone else in a position of trust with the opportunity—and the incentive— to exercise undue influence over the dependent party.

In some jurisdictions a presumption that undue influence was exercised arises whenever fiduciaries receive substantial benefits by gift or contract from their charges. However, it may be too harsh to apply a presumption that mechanically invalidates gifts or voids contracts between physicians and patients. The grateful patient is a real—if vanishing—phenomenon. Tangible expressions of gratitude should not be regarded routinely as the fruit of unconscionable behavior on the recipient's part. Each situation should be examined on its own to determine whether in fact the physician exercised undue influence in the property sense with respect to a particular patient.

The physician's fiduciary role as an advisor on questions of patient health is not at issue in these cases. Only if the facts demonstrate a special reason that the physician should be considered a fiduciary in the property sense should the law presume that substantial gifts or advantageous contracts unrelated to health care were procured through the exercise of undue influence. Such a finding might be appropriate when the patient was aged and infirm, or very young and impressionable, and no one else was interested in or responsible for the patient's financial well-being. It would not, however, be in order when the patient was mature and actively managing his or her own affairs. This is not to say that a competent adult could never be the victim of undue influence exercised by a physician. It simply means that the law should not presume the existence of undue influence—casting on physicians the burden of exonerating themselves—unless the circumstances dictate a particular reason for doing so.

With respect to physician involvement in for-profit medicine, the gift cases seem to have no particular relevance. The contract cases, however, are another matter. If a patient contracts with a physician's profit-making entity, such as a nursing home, for ancillary health care services, the law should scrutinize the contract very closely for evidence that the patient was not improperly persuaded to agree to its terms. Perhaps a presumption of undue influence might be appropriate under those circumstances, requiring the physician to prove that the patient entered freely into the contract. Certainly, when the terms of the contract appear unduly advantageous to the physician, courts ought to be particularly alert to possible breach of fiduciary duty.

Physician as Advisor

The second general category of fiduciaries concerns people who act as advisors and who are therefore in a position to exercise undue influence over what their charges do. The lawyer counseling a client is the strongest example, but the physician-patient relationship is strikingly similar. Both of these professionals often function in a dual capacity. They not only advise with respect to their patients' or clients' options but they themselves also often provide the very professional services they counsel their advisees to accept or reject. At the outset, therefore, they may be faced with a conflict between their advisees' best interests and their own financial well-being. That conflict is intensified when, for example, physicians stand to profit additionally from the ancillary services they advise their patients to consume because of their equity interest in the organization providing the services. This aspect of the physician's fiduciary obligation is seen in several types of cases.

Confidentiality Cases   The Hippocratic oath states "[w]hatever, in connection with my professional practice . . . I may see or hear . . . which ought not to be spoken abroad I will not divulge. . . ." For more than 2,000 years physicians have taken that oath, pledging themselves to secrecy with respect to confidential medical information. This self-assumed duty has fiduciary quality, for patients have no choice but to trust their medical advisors when they reveal the intimate details of their lives. Complete openness is often essential to effective treatment, but such one-sided honesty diminishes the patient's ability to deal with the physician on a basis of equality. The duty of confidentiality, springing originally from ethical principles, is designed to reinforce the relationship of trust between physician and patient in the interest of getting to the root of the patient's medical and emotional problems.[16]

In discussing breaches of medical confidentiality, some courts analyze the physician's duty as an implied provision of the physician-patient contract. That may well be true, but the force of the duty goes beyond mere contractual analysis. Physician-patient interaction does not necessarily involve contractual principles, yet no one would claim that lack of a contract gives a political candidate's physician license to broadcast that the patient is suffering from, for example, a terminal or even a social disease.

Recovery for breach of the duty of confidentiality is sometimes granted squarely on fiduciary grounds, the contract aside, because of the broader range of available remedies. Contract recovery generally is limited to economic loss occasioned by the breach, whereas equity encompasses a broader range of remedies. For example, equity can redress the mental distress and damage to a marital relationship that often accompany unauthorized disclosure of medical information, whereas damages for breach of contract would not.[17] Moreover, when physicians seek to disclose confidential medical information, courts can enjoin their behavior by citing fiduciary principles. Thus, when a psychiatrist published a book based on a thinly disguised account of a particular patient's therapy, a New York Supreme Court had no trouble enjoining its further distribution, as well as awarding damages, on the basis of a breach of fiduciary obligation.[18]

The confidentiality cases reinforce the concept of physicians as the guardians of their patients' total welfare. Although they are not always directly relevant to the issue of physician involvement in for-profit medical care, they demonstrate that injury to the patient's financial status can sometimes be as much the physician's responsibility as is the patient's medical condition or emotional state. Furthermore, when there is any suggestion that physicians are improperly using confidential medical information for personal gain, courts are quick to grant whatever redress is necessary to mitigate the damage caused by breach of the fiduciary relationship.

Statute of Limitations Cases   Another situation that raises the issue of the physician as fiduciary pertains to the applicable statute of limitations in medical malpractice cases. The law requires that at some point in time a patient's right to sue a doctor for malpractice must expire. Because memories fade, evidence is lost, and circumstances change with the passage of years, legislatures have passed statutes of limitation to govern the time period within which lawsuits must be brought. In some jurisdictions the date of the allegedly negligent act starts the limitations period running, although in others the discovery rule prevails (i.e., the statutory period begins with discovery of the injury). However, under a theory known as the continuous treatment doctrine, the cause of action will not accrue until the physician-patient relationship ends.[19]

The continuous treatment doctrine is based squarely on fiduciary considerations. It contemplates that patients can justifiably rely on their physician's good faith and professional ability during the course of the relationship. They are under no obligation to question the physician's techniques or to second guess opinions because they have a right to depend on the physician's fiduciary obligation to act solely in accordance with their best interests. Because physicians can cover up their mistakes during the continuation of treatment, they are not permitted to take advantage of a shorter limitations period during which they might have lulled the patient into a false sense of security or compromised the patient's ability to gain information about the true nature of his or her condition.

Here again the advisory role of the physician is the key to fiduciary responsibilities. The physician's dominance in the relationship is counterbalanced by special advantages granted to the patient by the law. Although the cases may not seem directly related to physician involvement in for-profit medicine, they highlight the fact that when a physician's self-interest conflicts with the patient's welfare, the law uses fiduciary theory to balance the scales in favor of the weaker party to the relationship.

Informed Consent Cases   Fiduciary aspects of the physician-patient relationship can also be seen in informed consent cases. The early informed consent opinions granted recovery to plaintiffs for unauthorized medical treatment on a battery rationale. If the patients had not consented to whatever procedures were performed, their physicians quite literally had trespassed upon their bodies. Over time, courts realized that such a simplistic analysis was not helpful in situations where patients had technically agreed to treatment but had not understood what their consent really meant. Informed consent cases thus came to be brought on the grounds of negligence rather than battery, on the theory that a physician's duty of care includes providing a certain level of information to the patient before proceeding with or abandoning treatment. The physician's special position of trust requires him or her to serve the patient's best interests, including the right to personal autonomy, above all else. Thus, the patient's consent will protect the physician only to the extent that the physician has not taken advantage of the fiduciary position to procure it.

The theory of recovery for failure to secure informed consent is grounded on the idea that, in the words of Mr. Justice Cardozo: "Every human being of adult years and sound mind has a right to determine what shall be done with his own body. . . ."[20] In other words, the decision maker is the patient not the physician. Unfortunately for this rationale, the physician usually understands the implications of medical information much better than the average patient.

This inequality of knowledge, however, is precisely what triggers the fiduciary aspect of the transaction. The physician has tremendous power over patients because the physician possesses the technical information and understands its implications. The physician also controls access to two things that may be critical to the patient's health: hospital admission and availability of prescription drugs. Moreover, the physician has great influence with respect to channeling sick people to appropriate specialists. The comparatively impotent patient approaches the physician for advice, with little choice but to trust that it will be given with the patient's best interests in mind. The additional conflict of interest raised when physicians derive secondary income from the care they advise their patients to accept can only impair that trust. It may not be necessary to eliminate such conflict altogether, but disclosure would at least counter the suspicion that secrecy is symptomatic of unethical behavior. If disclosure raises patients' doubts about recommended care because they know it would generate secondary income for their doctors, patients could seek second opinions on its necessity or seek care from a physician who does not have such conflict of interest.

Physician as Agent

The third category of fiduciaries deals with agents, i.e., persons who act for others in a representative capacity. As fiduciaries, agents are not permitted to take personal advantage of business opportunities that come their way in the course of service to their principals. For example, an agent cannot purchase property for him or herself that is offered for sale at an advantageous price to a principal whom the agent represents. By analogy, when physicians make certain decisions for their patients, perhaps they should only do so untainted by the conflict of interest that the receipt of secondary profits from their decisions would entail. Cases involving the physician's so-called therapeutic privilege to withhold information from patients in their own interest provide good examples of this aspect of physician as fiduciary.

So long as a patient is competent the major exception to the principle of patient self-determination with respect to medical treatment concerns the therapeutic privilege doctrine.[21] If a physician feels that a patient cannot deal psychologically with the truth about his or her medical condition or the treatment alternatives, therapeutic privilege permits the physician to adopt a paternalistic stance with regard to fact disclosure and decision making. In those relatively rare circumstances the patient's family acts as surrogate decision maker or, if family members are unwilling or unable to occupy that role, the physician may take on the decision-making function.

A physician acts as a fiduciary more in the agency than the advisory sense when preempting the patient's right to self-determination and preventing the patient from making decisions. The parallel to agency theory is not exact, because a true agent remains subject to the principal's commands. To the extent that a physician purports to act for the patient, however, the physician should be held to an agent's fiduciary standard of behavior. The physician can only justify depriving the patient of personal sovereignty if in the physician's professional opinion the patient's own best interests would otherwise be severely compromised. If the physician defends such drastic interference with the patient's fundamental right to self-determination on the grounds that the patient's best interests demand it, it should be obvious that any competing interests of the physician must be held to an irreducible minimum. If the exercise of therapeutic privilege were to be tainted by the physician's receipt of secondary income from treatment decisions the physician has made for the patient, a court might well find that this irreducible minimum has been exceeded.

There are other common physician-patient situations where fiduciary principles come into play, such as the human experimentation, right to die, and children's rights cases, but most of these in fact involve issues of informed consent. In addition, the physician's "fiduciary" duty toward society at large has been invoked in cases involving hospital staff privileges and the duty to warn third parties about potential harm from psychiatric patients.

It may be difficult to characterize some of these latter situations as involving the potential for conflict of interest in anything but an attenuated sense, but the use of fiduciary terminology to support the results reinforces the notion that the special societal status accorded physicians is accompanied by special responsibilities imposed by the judiciary. Legislatures can also impose special responsibilities, and one of the purposes of this paper is to stimulate thinking about whether that might be an advisable method for dealing with the conflict of interest presented by physician involvement in for-profit medical enterprises.

Conclusion

The foregoing discussion has traced development of the fiduciary principles applicable to physician-patient interaction, focusing on the way physicians have been considered fiduciaries in the property law sense, the advisory sense, and the agency sense. Although research has disclosed no cases directly raising fiduciary issues about physician involvement in the medical-industrial complex, an intriguing potential for liability exists.

A physician's receipt of secondary income from the services he or she recommends for a patient presents a potential conflict of interest with the patient's best interests. The conflict is intensified if we consider the physician a fiduciary on more than one basis when the physician advises a patient about treatment. In the first place the physician has fiduciary obligations arising out of the trust inherent in the role of advisor. Additionally, the physician might be considered a fiduciary in the property law sense because of the responsibilities toward the financial resources available for a patient's care. It is this intertwining of the advisory role with derivative power over the purse that exacerbates the potential for and seriousness of any abuse.

The law applicable to conflicts of interest generated by physician involvement in the medical-industrial complex is ripe for development. As noted previously, both the opportunity and the incentive for wrongful manipulation of the trust inherent in the physician-patient relationship are present. The issues may be resolved differently, however, depending on such factors as the percentage of the physician's ownership interest in a profit-making enterprise, the directness or indirectness of the secondary income benefit the physician receives, and the patient's ability to secure alternate forms of recommended treatment from other providers.

The content of the law that develops in this area will be affected by fiduciary theory, and a rather ironic development in a closely related area of the law probably will be influential as well. The Supreme Court has recently delivered several opinions facilitating antitrust litigation against the medical profession. By implication, these opinions damage the public perception of physicians as fiduciaries. Two decisions in particular, both rendered in the 1982 term, are especially relevant to the issue of physician involvement in for-profit medical care.

In *Arizona* v. *Maricopa County Medical Society*[22] the Supreme Court held that agreement among physicians on a schedule of maximum fees for health insurance reimbursement amounted to price fixing, illegal per se under the antitrust laws. The Court explicitly rejected the argument that the agreements should escape per se illegality categorization because they were entered into by medical professionals governed by ethical norms. On the facts of the case the Court refused to "distinguish the medical profession from any other provider of goods and services." In the other case, *Federal Trade Commission* v. *American Medical Association*,[23] the Court let stand a lower court finding that the AMA was organized to carry on business for the profit of its members.

These cases focus attention on the behavior of physicians as persons in commerce in apparent contradiction to their historic fiduciary image. The Supreme Court has expressly recognized that physicians can be influenced by the profit motive differentiated from pure professional concern for their patients' interests. In other words, the more physicians behave like ordinary businessmen, fixing prices and lobbying for financial interest through trade associations, the more the courts are going to treat them that way. On the other hand, the more they adhere to their disinterested fiduciary role, the less likely they arc to run afoul of laws designed to govern arm's-length commercial transactions. Perhaps a more stringent application of fiduciary principles to physician behavior might be in the best interests of the medical profession. In the long run, physicians might prefer to forego secondary income from the ancillary services they order for their patients if it reduces their overall exposure to liability. Their patients and society might benefit as well.

References and Notes

1. *Meinhard* v. *Salmon*, 164 N.E. 545, 546, (N.Y. 1928).

2. Relman, Arnold S., "The New Medical-Industrial Complex." *The New England Journal of Medicine* 303 (1980), p. 963.

3. The potential for *indirect* conflict of interest between physicians and patients exists when physicians are members of Blue Shield or other private health insurer governing boards, where they influence reimbursement policy and utilization review. When physicians have power to affect the fees they are paid or the procedures for which they are reimbursed from third parties, self-interest can collide with cost containment strategy. Whether driven by the technological imperative or by the desire to make more money, practicing physicians usually have little incentive to cut down on the amount of health care delivered or its cost. Physician dominance over hospital credentialling procedures presents another example of indirect conflict of interest. Physicians who control access to hospital privileges can protect their own incomes by preventing less expensive or more skilled physicians from competing for their patients.

These indirect financial conflicts of interest are in some sense unavoidable. Insurers depend on medical professionals for information about appropriate utilization, although the same may not be true with respect to price, because they lack the expertise to evaluate it themselves. Likewise, hospitals have little choice but to turn to medical professionals for ongoing assessment of a physician's clinical capability.

In the industrial and military medicine contexts, a physician's professional responsibility must be to the employee-patient unless the patient comes to the physician for an explicit evaluation of job fitness, even though the physician's salary is paid by a corporation or the government. The physician's relationship to his or her employer may present an indirect conflict of interest with the physician's duty to a patient by tempting the physician to pass on confidential medical information that could help the company but harm the patient's career. The law has a negative response to such breaches of the physician's fiduciary duty of confidentiality, however. A company or military physician occupies a unique position of divided loyalty in the corporate hierarchy, but legal doctrine acknowledges the conflict and defines appropriate behavior toward patients by focusing on the reason for the physician-patient interaction.

4. This paper is *not* concerned with the indirect conflicts of interest discussed in note 3, *supra*, nor is it concerned with *de minimus* conflicts of interest between physician and patient. Physician ownership of stock in a publicly traded drug company, for example, presents such a *de minimus* conflict. Even though a physician might prescribe the company's product for a patient, any impact on secondary income would be exceedingly remote.

5. Rettig, Richard A., "The Policy Debate on Patient Care Financing for Victims of End-Stage Renal Disease," *Law and Contemporary Problems* 40 (1976), p. 196.

6. Cf., Lowrie, Edmund G., and Hampers, C. L., "The Success of Medicare's End-Stage Renal-Disease Program," *The New England Journal of Medicine* 305 (1981) p. 434, which argues that freestanding, profit-making dialysis centers are more efficient and reduce costs.

7. Finn, P. D., *Fiduciary Obligation* (Sydney: The Law Book Co., 1977), p. 1.

8. Equity courts, as distinct from courts of law, extend jurisdiction where the remedy at law is inadequate or incomplete. Historically, the system of equity jurisprudence developed partly in response to the unwillingness or inability of common law courts to grant relief in trust cases where the beneficiary's rights had been violated. Most courts today, however, exercise both law and equity jurisdiction simultaneously. Although there is some overlap, the body of equity jurisprudence is still considered a separate entity from legal doctrine. Equity jurisdiction is invoked to provide relief where the legal remedy of money damages is either inappropriate or does not adequately redress the petitioner's grievance. Equitable remedies are usually more flexible than legal ones and are different in the sense that they can force one to *do* or *refrain from doing* something, as opposed to simply compensating the plaintiff for an injury.

9. A fourth category of fiduciary relationships, with few unifying themes to tie the cases together, serves as a catchall for certain other situations in which a court determines that a duty of loyalty has been breached or undue influence has been exercised and equity demands relief. For example, controlling shareholders have often been considered corporate fiduciaries, and franchisors have sometimes discovered to their dismay that they owe special obligations to their franchisees. Other remedies might have been available to the parties to these transactions, but the flexibility of equitable relief can make fiduciary categorization particularly attractive. See, generally, Talbott, Malcolm D., "Restitution Remedies in Contract Cases: Finding a Fiduciary or Confidential Relationship to Gain Remedies," *Ohio State Law Journal* 20 (1959), p. 320. This category is currently in the process of definition and expansion, as the law moves toward an unconscionable transaction theory of fiduciary obligation. See Shepherd, J. C., *The Law of Fiduciaries*, (Toronto: Carswell Co., 1981), p. 20. The trend has interesting implications for physician involvement in the medical-industrial complex, for it does not necessarily require evidence of bad faith to trigger a remedy.

10. *Forziati* v. *Board of Registration in Medicine*, 128 N.E.2d 789, 791 (Mass. 1955).

11. *Lilly* v. *Commissioner of Internal Revenue*, 188 F.2d 269, 271 (4th Cir. 1951). The Supreme Court reversed the case at 343 U.S. 90 (1952), but since the question at issue was the optical company's ability to take the kickbacks as an income tax deduction, the tax result does not necessarily undermine the fiduciary point.

12. "Pacemaker Investigations Charge Overuse and Corrupt Sales Practices." *Medical World News* (Sept. 1, 1982), p. 8.

13. But see, Pauly, Mark V., "The Ethics and Economics of Kickbacks and Fee Splitting," *Bell Journal of Economics* 10 (Spring 1979), p. 344, positing that fee splitting could in fact improve patient welfare.

14. Havighurst, Clark, "Controlling Health Care Costs: Strengthening the Private Sector's Hand," *Journal of Health Politics, Policy and Law* 1 (1976-1977), p. 471.

15. See, generally, Winder, W. H. D., "Undue Influence and Fiduciary Relationship," *The Conveyancer* 4 (March 1940), p. 274.

16. There may be situations, however, where the duty of confidentiality must yield to a higher societal interest. If psychiatrists reasonably believe patients present a significant risk of harm to themselves or to others, the duty of confidentiality is replaced by a duty to warn the appropriate authorities. *Tarasoff* v. *Regents of the University of California*, 551 P.2d 334 (Cal. 1976). Similarly, if a physician has reason to believe that a patient is the victim of child abuse or the carrier of a communicable disease, both the common law and statute may require the physician to report that fact. These cases where societal interests override the patient's right to confidentiality are clearly distinguishable from the ordinary situation wherein the patient simply confides in the physician for medical advice.

17. *MacDonald* v. *Clinger*, 84 App. Div. 482 (N.Y. 1982).

18. *Doe* v. *Roe*, 400 N.Y. Supp.2d 668 (1977).

19. *Stafford* v. *Shultz*, 270 P.2d 1 (Cal. 1954).

20. *Schloendorf* v. *Society of New York Hospital*, 105 N.E. 92, 129 (N.Y. 1912).

21. Meisel, Alan, "The Exceptions to the Informed Consent Doctrine: Striking a Balance Between Competing Values in Medical Decisionmaking," *Wisconsin Law Review* (1979), p. 413.

22. 50 U.S.L.W. 4687 (1982).

23. 50 U.S.L.W. 4313 (1982).

Biographical Sketches of Contributors

BRADFORD H. GRAY, Ph.D., is a senior professional associate at the Institute of Medicine. He was study director for the Institute studies *Access to Medical Review Data: Disclosure Policy for Professional Standards Review Organizations* (1981), *Health Care in a Context of Civil Rights* (1981), and *Evaluating Patient Package Inserts* (1979). The author of *Human Subjects in Medical Experimentation* (New York: Wiley-Interscience, 1975), he served on the staff of both the National Commission for the Protection of Human Subjects in Biomedical and Behavioral Research and the President's Commission for the Study of Ethical Problems in Medicine. Dr. Gray holds a Ph.D. in sociology from Yale University and taught at the University of North Carolina, Chapel Hill. He is currently the study director of the Institute of Medicine's study of physician involvement in for-profit enterprise in health care.

JOHN F. HORTY obtained his A.B. from Amherst College and his LL.B. from Harvard Law School. Mr. Horty is a member of the law firm of Horty, Springer & Mattern, president of Pittsburgh Planning Associates, Inc., both of Pittsburgh, Pennsylvania, and is counsel to the firm of Swidler, Berlin & Strelow, chartered, in Washington, D.C. He is the author and editor of two publications, *Action-Kit for Hospital Law* and *Action-Kit for Hospital Trustees*, and is author of *Patient Care Law*. He presently serves as president of the National Council of Community Hospitals, as chairman of the board of directors of Central Medical Center and Hospital

171

in Pittsburgh, and as a director and vice-president of Estes Park Institute. Mr. Horty is an honorary fellow of the American College of Hospital Administrators, a recipient of the Award of Honor of the American Hospital Association, and holds an honorary life membership in the American Hospital Association.

HAROLD S. LUFT, Ph.D., is professor of health economics, Institute for Health Policy Studies, University of California, San Francisco. His recent areas of research interest include health maintenance organizations, competition among hospitals, and multiple choice insurance arrangements. He is the author of *Health Maintenance Organizations: Dimensions of Performance* (New York: Wiley-Interscience) and with Joan Trauner and Joy Robinson has recently completed a monograph for the Federal Trade Commission, *Entrepreneurial Trends in Health Care Delivery: The Development of Retail Dentistry and Freestanding Ambulatory Services.*

FRANCES H. MILLER is professor of law at Boston University School of Law and has served in several health regulatory capacities in state government. Her writing in the health law field has focused on the potential for provider conflict of interest. See, for example, "Antitrust and the Certificate of Need: Health Systems Agencies, the Planning Act and Regulatory Capture," *Georgetown Law Journal* 68 (1980), p. 873; and "PSRO Data and Information: Disclosure to State Health Regulatory Agencies," *Boston University Law Review* 57 (1977), p. 245. She was recently named to a three-year Kellogg Foundation Fellowship that will enable her to study international health care delivery systems.

DANIEL M. MULHOLLAND III is a member of the law firm of Horty, Springer & Mattern, of Pittsburgh, Pennsylvania, which specializes in the practice of hospital and health care law. He also is a research editor for *Action-Kit for Hospital Law*, a monthly newsletter and treatise read nationwide. He has coauthored a number of articles in legal and hospital journals concerning the law as it relates to hospital chief executive officers, trustees, and medical staffs. Mr. Mulholland received his bachelor of arts and master of arts degrees from Duquesne University and his juris doctor degree from the University of Pittsburgh School of Law.

STEPHEN M. SHORTELL, Ph.D., is the A. C. Buehler distinguished professor of hospital and health services management and professor of organization behavior in the Department of Organization Behavior at the J. L. Kellogg Graduate School of Management, Northwestern University. He also holds appointments in the Department of Sociology and the Division of Community Medicine, School of Medicine, at Northwestern and formerly served as professor and chairman of the Department of Health Services, School of Public Health and Community Medicine, at the University of Washington, Seattle. Dr. Shortell received his undergraduate degree from the University of Notre Dame, his master's degree in public health and hospital administration from UCLA, and his Ph.D. in the behavioral sciences from the University of Chicago. He is the author of numerous articles and author or coauthor of several books and monographs, including *Organizational Research in Hospitals* and *Health Program Evaluation*. He serves on the editorial boards of several journals and is a consultant to a number of federal agencies, hospitals, and private foundations. He is currently conducting research on hospital-sponsored group practices and on hospital organizational responses to regulation.

RICHARD B. SIEGRIST, JR., is a project manager in the financial planning department at New England Medical Center in Boston. He holds an M.S. degree in accounting from New York University and a B.A. degree in political economy from Williams College. He is also a CPA and received his M.B.A. from Harvard Business School, where he wrote case studies on Hospital Corporation of America and Humana, Inc., for the Harvard Business School under the direction of Professor Regina E. Herzlinger.

JESSICA TOWNSEND has a degree in philosophy, politics, and economics from Oxford University, England. After a number of years as an economist and as a journalist for *Business Week*, she received a master's degree in health care administration from George Washington University and entered the field of health policy research. She subsequently participated in studies at the American Health Planning Association and the Institute of Medicine.

ROBERT M. VEATCH, Ph.D., is professor of medical ethics at the Kennedy Institute of Ethics, Georgetown University. He has training in pharmacology and obtained his doctorate in ethics from Harvard University. His research work is primarily in ethics and health policy. Dr. Veatch's books include *A Theory of Medical Ethics* and *Case Studies in Medical Ethics*. He is co-editor of the collection *Ethics and Health Policy*.

Index

A

accreditation of hospitals, 19
administrators, *see* hospital, administrators
advertising, medical profession, 7, 127–128
American Hospital Association *Guide*, 52
American Medical Association (AMA)
  code of ethics, 6–7, 126–128, 130–134, 138, 145
  v. *Federal Trade Commission*, 167
  views on patents, 128
  views on physician advertising, 128
  views on physician ownership of health care facilities, 130–132
American Medicorp, 46–47
American Osteopathic Association, 19
Arizona v. *Maricopa County Medical Society*, 166–167

B

boards of directors, 18, 44, 88
  of for-profit hospitals, 136
  of nonprofit hospitals, 20–21
  open meetings of, 29–30
  quality of care and, 22
Brookwood Health Services, 46, 47

C

capital costs
  bond financing, 26, 28
certificate of need (CON) legislation, 43, 53, 58, 64
code of ethics
  American Bar Association, 137–138
  American Medical Association, 6–7, 126–1228, 130–134, 138, 145
  Australian Medical Association, 127
  British Medical Association, 127
  certified public accountants, 136
  engineers, 137
  physicians' compared with those of other professionals, 136–138
  see also ethics; medical ethics

175